Gut Wellness Simplified

Exploring the Unseen Universe
Within Us

Olivia Rivers

© **Copyright 2023 - All rights reserved.**

The content contained within this book may not be reproduced, duplicated, or transmitted without direct written permission from the author or the publisher.

Under no circumstances will any blame or legal responsibility be held against the publisher, or author, for any damages, reparation, or monetary loss due to the information contained within this book, either directly or indirectly.

Legal Notice:

This book is copyright protected. It is only for personal use. You cannot amend, distribute, sell, use, quote or paraphrase any part, or the content within this book, without the consent of the author or publisher.

Disclaimer Notice:

Please note the information contained within this document is for educational and entertainment purposes only. All effort has been executed to present accurate, up to date, reliable, complete information. No warranties of any kind are declared or implied. Readers acknowledge that the author is not engaged in the rendering of legal, financial, medical, or professional advice. The content within this book has been derived from various sources. Please consult a licensed professional before attempting any techniques outlined in this book.

By reading this document, the reader agrees that under no circumstances is the author responsible for any losses, direct or indirect, that are incurred as a result of the use of the information contained within this document, including, but not limited to, errors, omissions, or inaccuracies.

Kick Start Your Gut Wellness Journey!

Enjoy our 7-day Gut-Healing Meal Plan to jumpstart your transformative journey to vibrant gut health, including a shopping list for your convenience.

Simply scan the QR code and follow the instructions to access your downloadable PDF. It's quick, easy, and ready to empower your well-being!

Embark on a flavorful, nourishing adventure toward gut wellness. Fuel your body with wholesome recipes and embrace the joy of prioritizing your digestive health.

Here's to your vibrant, thriving gut and a journey filled with nourishment and vitality!

Table of Contents

INTRODUCTION 1

CHAPTER 1: UNDERSTANDING THE GUT 7
    THE GUT: ITS PARTS AND PROBLEMS 8
        Esophagus 8
    THE GUT-BRAIN AXIS 14

CHAPTER 2: THE GUT AND OVERALL WELL-BEING 17
    GUT HEALTH AND WEIGHT 17
    GUT HEALTH AND IBS 19
    GUT HEALTH AND HEART HEALTH 21
    DIABETES AND GUT HEALTH 23
    UNHEALTHY GUT: KNOW THE SIGNS 24

CHAPTER 3: CUMULATIVE EFFECTS—GUT HEALTH AND GENDER 29
    ANIMAL STUDIES 30
    HUMAN STUDIES 32
    SEX HORMONES 33
    DIET 35
    DRUGS 36
    DISEASE 37

CHAPTER 4: WOMEN AND GUT HEALTH 41
    TUMMY TROUBLES 42
    HORMONES 43
    NUTRITION FOR WOMEN 46
    BAD FOODS: STAY AWAY! 49

CHAPTER 5: BALANCING THE GUT—THE GUT CLEANSE 55
    WHY SHOULD WE DO A CLEANSE? 56
    METHODS FOR CLEANING YOUR DIGESTIVE SYSTEM 57
    SIDE EFFECTS 61
    THE COFFEE ENEMA 63

 The Alleged Benefits of the Coffee Enema 64
 The Research 65

CHAPTER 6: MENTAL HEALTH AND THE GUT 69
 HOW ARE THE GUT AND BRAIN CONNECTED? 70
 MENTAL HEALTH AND INFLAMMATION 71
 PROBIOTICS 72
 MENTAL HEALTH STRATEGIES 73
  Staying Connected 74
  Exercise 75
  Learning New Skills 76
 MENTAL HEALTH IN AMERICA 78

CHAPTER 7: EATING FOR YOUR GUT—THE ROLE OF DIET AND EXERCISE 83
 PROTEIN 85
 FATS 86
 CARBS 87
  Digestible Carbs 87
  Non-Digestible Carbs (Fiber) 88
 PROBIOTICS 89
 EXERCISE 91
  Sample Exercises for Gut Health 93
  Machines 97

CHAPTER 8: MYTHS AND TRUTHS—FAQS 101
 MYTH #1: YOU SHOULD POOP EVERY DAY 101
 MYTH #2: STRESS CAUSES STOMACH ULCERS 103
 MYTH #3: ALL BACTERIA ARE BAD FOR US 105
 MYTH #4: GLUTEN IS BAD FOR YOUR GUT 107
 MYTH #5: [INSERT FAD DIET HERE] WORKS! 110
 MYTH #6: CHEWING GUM WILL SIT IN YOUR STOMACH FOR 7 YEARS 112
 MYTH #7: EATING BEFORE BED IS BAD FOR YOU 118
 MYTH #8: "LEAKY GUT" RESULTS IN FOOD PARTICLES ENTERING YOUR BLOODSTREAM 121

CONCLUSION **125**

ADDITIONAL RESOURCES **133**
  BOOKS 133
  ARTICLES 134
  WELLNESS EXPERTS 134

REFERENCES **137**

Introduction

"Gut" is a fantastic word. It reminds me of childhood, where you might hear kids say someone was "punched in the gut," for example, because "stomach" and "tummy" were considered baby-like. There was also the great song about "greasy, grimy gopher guts," which, while disgusting, comes attached to memories of campfires and that ecstatic feeling of saying something taboo.

There is also the verb, obviously: "to gut." We use this when we take out the innards of a fish or some game we shot on a hunting trip. It has the connotation, then, of being something disgusting. It is just transgressive enough to feel icky and slimy. Which is probably why, as kids, it was always associated with being slightly more grown up: It meant you could conjure up something gross instead of something safe and sanitary. "Tummy" was not a good descriptor because it seemed nice.

"Gut" was gross in the way a word like "fart" was better than "passing gas." Gross enough for kids to know it sounds adult and for adults to know it sounds like something for kids. After all, at a certain point, we stop trying to be gross and instead just try to be accurate.

This is why it is funny to me to hear medical professionals and health experts refer to "gut health." It sounds at first like maybe this or that health expert is still stuck in some kind of perpetual infanthood.

Do medical professionals not have fancier words than "gut?" Are we still trying to be gross instead of being accurate, adults—grown up?

What I am trying to say here is that you should not be fooled by the concept of the "gut." Whatever it sounds like to you, however, fifth grade or whatever else, this is one of the sneakily most important parts of our body. It has connections to all sorts of areas of our well-being.

And we are going to use it to unlock the secrets of healthy living.

As it turns out, our digestive system, or "gut," is just as, if not more, complex than we could have ever thought. It covers an enormous array of organs and travels an enormous length, all wrapped up inside our bodies. And within that are all sorts of microscopic entities, from viruses and bacteria to cells and all sorts of other things. All of these are working in tandem to ensure the safe passage of food, and all need to be kept in balance in order to ensure our continued good health.

As you may have heard, our bodies are not just a singular entity. Each body is made up of smaller and smaller parts, each of which is essential to its maintenance.

We have the ability, through poor food and exercise choices, to throw off this delicate balance. And if we do that, we suffer the downstream consequences, including, but not limited to, illness, lethargy, and brain fog.

Which means that keeping these things in balance can do just the opposite of that.

And that is what we are going to learn how to do.

Now, I said the body is not just a singular entity, and that is true. But the reality is that it is much more complicated than that.

See, our bodies are both parts and a whole. We have things like arms and legs, individual organs, and, as we said, the individual viruses and bacteria that live inside of us. All of these things are parts and can be, theoretically, removed.

The problem, of course, is that together they make up a whole. That "whole" is called "our body" and requires all of these individual things to be in working order so that they can function well.

When one thing is thrown off, there are problems that arise downstream of it. This is why, when talking about health, we need to talk about things both individually and holistically.

The gut is no different. The gut is a thing—a distinct system from the rest of the body. But the gut is still a part of the larger body. Its healthiness is not limited to itself, but instead, when it becomes unhealthy, a whole host of problems show up, many of them in bodily systems we might be accustomed to thinking of as distinct from the rest of the body.

This is something we are going to learn to rethink. As we are going to see, the health of the whole system is important and can only be thought of in terms of the health of its parts, all of which add up to the whole.

Which, I know, sounds kind of complicated. But it is not! In fact, before we are through here, I think we will have learned exactly how to think like this, in addition to lots of other things.

And what are those other things? Well, by the end of this book, we will have learned what the gut is, specifically, and how it works. We will have learned why it is so important to have a healthy gut and what it means to talk about a "microbiome."

We will have learned that our gut health is connected to all sorts of things. Our mental health, in addition to our physical health, is in some sense dependent upon maintaining a healthy gut microbiome. And in learning about this, we will unlock the secrets to healthy living through gut health.

But that is not all! We are going to cover how this is different for both men and women and how our hormones play a role in all of this. We are going to talk about cleanses, how gut health can help you manage depression symptoms, and how it can go the other way, too: Namely, that managing our mental health can also help promote good gut health.

And finally, we are going to talk about diet and exercise, the myths about gut health, and what you can and should do to keep that in good standing after you are done reading this book.

And we are going to do this using the best science we have at our disposal. As best as we can, we are going to stay away from junk and pseudoscience, away from cure-all claims and fad diet advice. We are going to stick to what is true, what matters, and what you can do to get the results you want.

In other words, we are going to send you on a path that, if you take it seriously, can make you strong, make you feel good, and help make you into the version of yourself you have always wanted to be.

Of course, these are lofty claims. But hopefully, by the time this book is through, you will have seen that not only are these results possible, but you, yourself, are more than capable of pulling this off.

So, with all that said, let us strap in, get comfortable, and keep an open and interested mind. We are going to be covering a lot of ground, but in the end, it will all be worth it.

So let us go, then, and begin the journey toward understanding gut health.

Chapter 1:
Understanding the Gut

"So, what," you might be asking, "is the gut, exactly? I know you said it was the digestive system, but what is that?"

Well, this is an excellent question. And good on you for asking, because too often we forget that it is always important to start with definitions. At least that way, we know where our ground is—our jumping-off point.

There are a few synonyms at work here: "gut," "digestive system," and "gastrointestinal tract." This encompasses everything from our mouth down to our anus, meaning the whole passageway through which food is processed, sent out to the rest of our bodies, and converted into energy.

The process begins, obviously, with chewing the food, which is broken down by saliva and then swallowed. Other than chewing and swallowing, however, the rest of our digestion is done involuntarily. We have no control over what happens inside our stomachs or in our intestines. These processes happen totally without our conscious input.

Which, yes, I know, everyone learns about in, like, first grade. But think about how amazing that is! We do not have to put a single thought into what happens in our small intestine, for example, and yet it happens anyway. Bodies are crazy.

But how many individual organs are taking part in this process? What are the different pieces of our digestive system, working essentially of their own accord?

Let's get to know them here.

The Gut: Its Parts and Problems

Esophagus

This is a hollow tube in your throat, a muscle that brings food and liquid down into your stomach. Notice that this is part of your digestive system, but it is right up against the trachea, which is part of your respiratory system. Rumor has it that we are one of the only animals who can choke, and this is why!

Stomach

Who does not know what the stomach is? This is where the food goes to be broken down by stomach acid. Food usually sits here between two and eight hours, although sometimes longer or shorter if you are having stomach issues. This is probably what we think of first when we think about the "gut."

Liver

One of the most remarkable organs in the body, the liver filters toxins out of your body in addition to producing bile. It has the ability to regenerate if parts of it are removed, and, given the amount of toxins we put into our body, it can really withstand a beating.

"Hepatitis" is the state in which your liver is inflamed, and cirrhosis is when it is permanently scarred or damaged beyond repair. That usually happens when you drink way too much or for a long period of time.

Gallbladder

When your liver produces bile, this is where it goes. The gallbladder releases bile as necessary. Removal of the gallbladder is a common surgery, usually due to stones or cancer.

Pancreas

This sweet Susie produces insulin! Your blood sugar goes up or down depending on whether you have just eaten, and how much it goes up or down is dependent on what and how much you have eaten. Your pancreas releases insulin in order to adjust your blood sugar and keep it from reaching dangerous levels.

Small intestine

This part of the digestive system absorbs the nutrients from the food or liquids you have consumed. It also continues the process of breaking down food, which is about to get considerably more disgusting.

Large intestine

Yep, here it comes. In this organ, you have billions of bacteria, which help turn food into feces. (Gross.) Water and electrolytes are also removed from the food, which the body will use for its own purposes.

Rectum

This part is right at the tail end of the large intestine. It is basically a temporary storage facility for feces right before it is released into the toilet, out in the woods, or wherever you are about to do your business.

Anus

And there it is—the butt.

This is the organ through which feces are expelled. Specifically, it is the outside part, in case you were wondering.

And this concludes the tour of the key parts of our digestive system. The takeaway here is that, as a system, it is both whole and in parts, and each of those parts has a specific function. Effectively, they are all there to take the food you put into your body, extract from that food the bits we need to live, and then expel what we do not need in the form of feces.

That we rely so much on billions of bacteria, specifically in the large intestine, is kind of remarkable. Organisms that are not us nonetheless live inside of us and rely on us for sustenance as much as we rely on them. Life, as they say, is pretty crazy.

Now, there are more things we could talk about in terms of specific areas of our digestive system. But for now, I would like to pivot over to the kinds of things that can go wrong with our digestion.

One of the most common is called "indigestion," which is the pain you get in your stomach when you are having trouble digesting food or fluids. "Heartburn" is a related condition, but much more specific.

Indigestion can suck—big time. The pain of indigestion can be so bad, in fact, that it can require people to lie down and wait for the moment to pass. But, alas, Pepto Bismol remains the best cure in the world for this particular ailment.

We are also all familiar with diarrhea. This is an utter ordeal of a thing in which feces are excreted in extraordinary amounts, with an alarming frequency, and mostly in a liquid form. Also known as "the squirts," in case you were wondering.

There are many things that cause diarrhea, so we will not get into them here. For now, we can mark this as one of the symptoms that something in our gut has been misaligned and is in need of fixing.

On the opposite end of the spectrum is constipation. This, for those who have never endured its particular brand of suffering, is when discharging feces (commonly called "pooping") becomes nigh-impossible or extremely difficult.

Common symptoms of this include bloating and nausea. Frequently, this is caused by not consuming enough fiber or, more often than not, too much cheese.

There is also a mean, demonic condition known as "food poisoning." If you have never had this, consider yourself lucky. Effectively, this happens when you have eaten something that has gone "bad," meaning it has some kind of bacterium on it that is causing your digestive system to go haywire.

This can produce a whole array of symptoms, each one more devious than the last. Fevers, chills, and diarrhea you would have never thought possible are all manifestations of this horror, which can only be solved by drinking lots of water and waiting for it to run its vile course.

Okay, so what was the point of all that?

Simply put, when your digestive system experiences a problem, you often experience it in ways that you wish you had not. The symptoms of digestive problems are almost always brutal and, at the very least, produce a profound sense of discomfort. At the most, which is not often, they can require hospitalization.

Taking care of this, then, is of paramount importance. Because nobody wants to let this slide and spend the whole day on the toilet. Nobody.

So, with all that in mind, we should get moving on the next big topic in this book: The microbiome.

The Microbiome: Everything We Need to Get Ourselves Started

First off, what is it?

Well, as we have already discussed, our body is filled with literally trillions of microorganisms, ranging from bacteria to viruses to even fungi. These organisms, which are known as "microorganisms," are not of the harmful type that we often encounter in the wild but are enormously beneficial to our health. Taken together, they are what is known as the microbiome.

It really is like an unseen universe within us!

In fact, and this is the crazy part, the human organism is actually made up of more bacteria cells than what we might call "human cells." The human body, in other words, is its own ecosystem, a universe of tiny things all working in tandem, each one benefiting the other and vice versa.

As regards its role, it might actually be beneficial to think of it as another organ. We have evolved over millions of years to survive with the help of the microbiome, so much so that without it, there is a good to fair chance we would not be able to survive at all (Robertson, 2023).

And this starts super early! Our first exposure to microbes happens when we exit the birth canal, although there is actually some evidence to suggest that our first interactions with them occur inside the womb. You then accumulate microbes as you grow older, to the point where your microbiome diversifies and takes on new functions. The higher the activity of your microbiome, the better (Robertson, 2023).

But where exactly do you interact with microbes out in the wild? Well, the food you eat has a huge role in this. And this plays a huge role early on, too: As a baby, you rely on microbes in your large intestine to break down the healthy sugars in breast milk. These are important for growth (Robertson, 2023).

Fiber, too, which is indigestible plant matter, is broken down by microbes, which then create short-chain fatty acids, which are important for gut health. Fiber, too, is one of the key ingredients to staving off weight gain, in addition to a whole host of other things, like heart disease (Robertson, 2023).

Here is another one that may surprise you: Your gut microbiome affects your immune system!

How this happens is that your gut microbiome responds to information in the gut, communicates with your immune cells, and thereby helps prevent infection (Robertson, 2023). It is quite different from what we consider when we think about having bacteria in our digestive system.

And finally, there is some evidence to show that your gut microbiome affects your central nervous system, which is then responsible for brain health (Robertson, 2023).

And that is not all—in fact, there is a deep connection between our brain and our gut. So much so that it even has a name: The gut-brain axis!

The Gut-Brain Axis

The first place to start is with neurons.

Now, we all know what these are. These are in our brains and nervous systems, and they more or less tell our bodies how to behave. The number of individual neurons in our brains is to the tune of 100 billion (Robertson, 2023).

But what about our guts? Well, as it turns out, there are 500 million neurons in our guts, which connect the gut to the brain. The vagus nerve is the name of the main nerve that connects our guts to our brains, and it is super important. For example, in animal studies, it has been found that stress actually interferes with the vagus nerve, which is why stress causes gastrointestinal problems.

And that is not all!

Neurotransmitters also connect the gut to the brain. These are chemicals that are produced in the brain and control our feelings and emotions. Serotonin is one of the more famous ones, and it is the one that contributes to our feelings of happiness and well-being.

In fact, this is why drugs like MDMA cause us to feel intense feelings of love, empathy, and happiness: They basically unleash an army of serotonin into our brains.

But here is an interesting thing: Serotonin is also produced in the gut, as is GABA, which controls our feelings of fear and anxiety.

So, all these trillions of microbes and neurotransmitters in our gut have an effect on our brain. Having things go awry in the gut can mean inducing feelings like stress and anxiety, or it might just flat-out interfere with our sense of general well-being.

Taking care of our gut, then, can mean increasing our feelings of happiness, in addition to all those others listed above. Our body, again, is holistic, an interconnected network of various things, all of which work together and affect one another.

What we can do to take care of our brains *via* our guts is going to be discussed in detail later. But for now, let us think for a second about how interesting that is and what the possibilities might be as far as our mental health if we just do something as simple as taking care of our gut health.

***

All in all, then, this unseen universe within us is insanely important for a whole host of different reasons. We have a gazillion things working away inside of us to keep us healthy, keep our immune system running smoothly, help us digest food in ways that benefit us, and keep our brains functioning.

We owe an enormous debt of gratitude to these things. Because, as we can see, we are kind of boned without them. So, how do we repay this debt?

By taking care of it, of course. Which is precisely what we are going to learn how to do!

With that in mind, then, it is time to take a deeper dive into what exactly we intend to do. We need to figure out just what we mean when we say that taking care of our gut health means increasing our well-being. And we need to look at specific case studies that suggest that this is not just mere conjecture or another one of those diet fads we are talking about here.

So, let's move on!

Chapter 2:
The Gut and Overall Well-Being

Now, I know what you are thinking: "Here we go, another diet writer speaking in generalizations, not giving me any specifics. Just what the heck happens to our health when we take care of our guts? And you'd better be specific—or else!"

First off, I do not respond to threats, so if I were you, I would take it down a notch. But nonetheless, I understand your concern. Lots of broad claims are made all the time about all sorts of things, and generally, they are a way of weaseling out of having to make claims that can be tested. Being specific just means being upfront and honest about what you are saying.

But really, if you had just been more patient, you would have seen that your anger is ill-founded, considering this entire chapter is dedicated to the health benefits downstream of caring for our gut microbiome. So, I don't know; maybe next time, wait a second. I mean, jeez...

Anyway, here are a few of the things we can link gut health to, in no particular order:

Gut Health and Weight

We know now that there are a whole slew of microbes in our guts, many of which are responsible for keeping us healthy. But in addition to that, and as we can imagine, there are unhealthy microbes that live in our guts as well. And when they get out of balance—a phenomenon sometimes known as dysbiosis—this can lead to unwanted weight gain (Robertson, 2023).

One study involved transplanting fecal microbiota from a pair of adult twins—one of whom was obese while the other was not—into germ-free, low-fat mouse chow, as well as food that was high in saturated fats and more in line with what we would understand as the typical American diet. According to the results, mice that consumed the fecal culture of the obese twin gained more weight than mice that consumed the same diet but without the obese twin's fecal culture in their food (Ridaura *et al.*, 2013).

Which is disgusting, yes. But consider what this means! The microbes present in an obese person's fecal matter—which, if you remember, means microbes in the large intestine—appear to have led to obesity when transferred into another organism, *no matter the diet they were consuming*. In other words, microbes themselves are a contributing factor with regard to someone becoming obese or not.

Or so it happens in mice. This is obviously not a one-to-one causal relationship, but it is interesting and worth thinking about.

This could mean that one way to control weight gain is to pay close attention to our gut health. And as if that were not cool enough in itself...

Gut Health and IBS

You read that correctly: There is good reason to believe that the cramping, bloating, and discomfort you may or may not be getting from IBS could be a result of an imbalance in your gut microbiome.

Now, why is this?

Well, one of the things about all those microbes is that they actually produce an awful lot of gas. This occurs as a result of the metabolic processes of the microbiota in your colon, although some air is brought into your gut as a result of swallowing. We are all quite familiar with the burping phenomenon, which is how our body reaches homeostasis after ingesting too much air. In addition to this, your small intestine theoretically also produces a certain amount of CO_2 when acids and alkalis are broken down (Campbell, 2020).

And yet, on top of the swallowing of air and the CO_2 that might be released in the small intestine, there are still those lingering gases produced by the microbiota. In the colon, this is a result of "colonic fermentation," which is where the gassy residues produced as a result of microbiotic metabolism become the substrates for those same microbiota. Essentially, the microbes produce the gas that they need in order to remain alive and in your colon.

So far, this is all normal and would not be considered sufficient to account for IBS. The problem is that some people are extra sensitive to the amount of gas in their digestive system and make this problem worse by consuming substances called "flatulogenic" or "fart-inducing." (I didn't make that up. That's an actual word.) When this happens, gas is produced at much higher levels than normal, which affects those with sensitive guts much more and may cause all kinds of discomfort, bloating, and other not-fun symptoms.

How do we know this? Well, apparently, when sufferers are given low-residue diets or diets that do not make them fart as much (seriously), the pain and discomfort abate. Which might suggest that this is an easy fix to the problem, but actually, it comes with a downside.

The problem is that the microbiota need that gaseous substrate in order to survive. And a low-residue diet, since it produces, by its nature, much less gas in the body, actually reduces the microbes in your colon.

This is obviously not a healthy choice. So, where does the solution lie?

As it turns out, using prebiotics might help. Apparently, during the first few days of using them, people with IBS will develop much worse symptoms but will undergo adaptation after a certain amount of time has passed. Once this happens, the microbiota will have started using the prebiotics as its substrate because they are fermented and then produce less gas during its normal fermentation process.

Yes, we are getting a bit ahead of ourselves here. The point I am making is that the microbiome is intimately tied to problems with intestinal gas, and dealing with it in a way that alters the number of microbes in our colon has further negative effects on our health.

In other words, the microbiome is a culprit when it comes to irritable bowel syndrome because the microbiome is so directly linked to intestinal health.

But wait—there's more!

Gut Health and Heart Health

As it turns out, the heart is one of the first things to get affected when you make all kinds of healthy or unhealthy dietary and lifestyle choices. This organ, not surprisingly, is really at the center of all things for us. And so, it should not be surprising that gut health directly impacts the healthiness of our hearts.

Now, that said, this is the science we are talking about—there are going to be divergent points of view on this, and many studies will seem to provide evidence for a multitude of different options. Being a good scientist often means being in a state of skepticism, where we understand that results can be influenced by all kinds of factors, that human beings are not perfect instruments for discerning the truth, and that a positive or negative result, even after being peer-reviewed and accepted by the scientific community at large, really only entitles us to a justified true belief, not a dogmatic acceptance of what we think of as fact.

So, with that in mind, the question we should be asking is less, "Does gut health directly influence heart health?" but rather,

"Are there signals that suggest that caring for our gut health means having healthier hearts as a result?"

And yes, there are, in fact, signals that seem to suggest exactly that.

One study from 2015 was interested in finding out if gut microbiota contributed to variations in body mass index and blood lipid levels ("lipid" being a fatty acid) among individuals. A discussion of the method by which they did this is beyond the scope of this book, but the participants numbered 893, which is, as you might have guessed, a lot of people but not an enormous amount (Fu *et al.*, 2015).

The results of this study showed that gut microbiota contributed to variations in BMI and lipid levels independent of age, sex, and genetics. Meaning those microbes in your digestive system can make anyone of any age, sex, or genetic predisposition overweight and have high fatty acid counts in their blood.

And what does this mean for heart health? Well, as we said, the heart is often one of the first things affected by diet and lifestyle choices. Being overweight, as it turns out, does quite a number on your cardiac system.

And those lipids we were talking about? That is what builds up plaque in your arteries, which leads to heart attacks. So, when your gut microbiome gets out of whack, you wind up setting the stage for a future heart attack, even if you are young, female, and have no family history of heart disease.

So, yes, you want a healthy heart? Take care of your digestion. And hey, while we are here, why don't we talk about...

Diabetes and Gut Health

That is right; up next, we have the ever-dependable diabetes. A prevalent disease that, as we all know, has to do with how our body regulates its blood sugar. Type 1 diabetes is an autoimmune disorder, but type 2 is caused by diet and lifestyle choices. Neither of them is fun to have, and both of them, therefore, should be avoided if and when possible.

But how does gut health tie into this?

Well, to begin with, a study of 33 infants, all of whom were predisposed to T1D, found some interesting correlations between their gut microbiomes and the onset of the disease. Basically, the subjects who developed T1D underwent a drop-off period before the disease manifested, in which the diversity of microbes declined. In other words, right before they developed T1D, they had fewer types of microbes in their guts than they did normally (Kostic *et al.*, 2015).

And not only that, but the number of *unhealthy* bacteria increased during that period. So, the healthy ones were the ones that went away.

Now, does this mean that it is possible to stave off the onset of T1D by ensuring bacterial diversity in the digestive system? Not necessarily. In fact, just what that means with regard to the prevention of the disease is about as clear as mud.

To begin with, this establishes correlation, but not causation. By this, I mean that we know, if only based on this one study, that the event "Decline in Bacterial Diversity in the Gut

Microbiome" precedes the event "Onset of T1D." Do we know that one causes the other? No. Something else, obviously, could be causing both of them. Or maybe there is some other, completely different explanation for why they seem to occur one after the other. That information is just not available to us in this study.

But there does seem to be some connection, right? Even with our skeptics' hats on, is this not at least kind of interesting?

And if, by the way, there does prove to be a causal relationship, is it possible that caring for our gut health might help prevent T1D in people who are already predisposed? Alas, this is not information we have either. But as a line of inquiry, there is no doubt that it appears to be worth pursuing. After all, T1D stinks, and anything we can do to prevent it from occurring is for the good.

Because that's the thing about diabetes, there really is nothing you can do to sugarcoat it.

Now, all of this is well and good. But what about those of us without diabetes, heart conditions, or weight problems? How do we know when we have an unhealthy gut? What are some of the signs that something has gone wrong?

Unhealthy Gut: Know the Signs

The specifics around each of these are going to be delved into later, rest assured. For now, we are going to do an overview so that we know *there are certain signs that our gut health is out of whack.*

And just what are those signs?

Well, remembering that it is our guts we are talking about, our stomach is going to be a decent guide as to whether or not our guts are in working order (Dix *et al.*, 2023). So, if we are having gut troubles, we will probably notice things like an upset stomach, bloating, or diarrhea. Maybe we have heartburn and do not have a condition that makes heartburn a regular occurrence.

A sudden, unintentional change in our weight might also be an indication that our guts are out of order. And this could go either way too: We could gain *or* lose weight, and either could be a symptom of this problem.

Experiencing sleep problems? Well, that too could be a symptom! Although the exact mechanism by which this occurs is still unknown, it might have something to do with the way our gut health interacts with our immune system. And it is for that reason that conditions like psoriasis might be made worse by poor gut health.

And since our gut bacteria are responsible, at least in part, for breaking down certain foods, if you develop a sudden food intolerance, it may come down to your gut health too. Lactose, for example, requires a specific kind of bacterium to be digested, and a lack of it might make you more susceptible to those pesky stomach issues that come with not tolerating milk super well.

You can also recognize that you are at risk of poor gut health based on your stress levels, how well you sleep, and what your diet is like. For example, a diet that is high in processed sugar, coupled with someone who is undersleeping and is next door to having a heart attack with stress every day, almost certainly has something wrong with their gut.

So, yeah. There are plenty of signs that things might have gone wrong and plenty of signs that things might go wrong in the future.

***

Where does this leave us?

While we have hinted at the kind of things we can do to keep our gut microbiome in working order, the main takeaway from this chapter, I think, is that this unseen universe in our digestive system packs a wallop in terms of its impact.

And really, why should it not? We have evolved to house these things and be their ecosystem.

Think of any old ecosystem as a comparative: Say, the Amazon. The Amazon houses something like three million different species including thousands of species of plants. Every one of these creatures and plants is dependent on all of the others, even if not always in a proximate way. Taking one out of the equation, then, causes serious damage for others.

Want an example? Okay, of all the animals that live in the rainforest, the worst of all of them is undoubtedly the Goliath bird-eating spider. How do I know this? Well, this beast of a thing is roughly the size of a dinner plate, which is terrifying. And, true to its name, it is known to eat hummingbirds. This means it is enormous and terrifying in equal measure, considering that most of the time, it is spiders who are eaten by birds.

As you can tell, I think this is a wretched thing. I *hate* the bird-eating spider. Purely as a reflex, if given the opportunity to eliminate all traces of this foul creature, my knee-jerk reaction would be to say, "Yes, of course. Get rid of it."

But what would happen if the bird-eater were to disappear without leaving a trace of its existence behind? In addition to occasionally eating birds, it also eats rodents. The rodent population, then, would begin to grow. Rodents eat bugs and vegetation, which means there would be fewer of both of those. And while eventually nature would adapt to this newfound disequilibrium, for a period, there would be chaos and adjustment.

Even the most disgusting among us is there for a reason. And that reason keeps everything working in a kind of harmony.

So, what is it with the bacteria, viruses, and fungi in our digestive tracts? We depend on them because we have evolved to house them and thereby live for mutual benefit.

And much like in nature, when that equilibrium is thrown off—say, when the bacteria we need become outnumbered by the ones that cause us harm—our vital functions begin to suffer as a result.

In essence, this book is not, by the looks of things, going to lead us astray. Gut health is a key ingredient in our overall functioning, and so taking care of it is only going to unlock a whole host of benefits.

And yet, no two bodies are the same. And humans, as a sexually dimorphic species, have different health requirements based on the sex of the body we are talking about.

So, before we get into the specifics as far as what we need to keep our guts healthy, let's dig into how gut health differs between men and women to make sure we are adequately prepared for recommendations regarding diet and exercise.

Chapter 3:
Cumulative Effects—Gut Health and Gender

Alright, this is going to be a challenging one. But we are going to get through it.

Firstly, I should mention that I know this is a sensitive topic. So, for clarification, we should start by saying that, as we have heard many, many times by now, sex and gender are two different categories. By "gender" we mean cultural expectations around behaviors associated with biological sex. And by "sex," then, we mean a biological category, as implied in the previous sentence. "Sex" is defined by gamete size, meaning testes indicate a male and ova indicate a female.

For the purposes of this chapter, we are going to be talking about biology; therefore, we are talking about sex, not gender.

But why is this important?

Male and female bodies react differently to the same stimuli. In large part, this is because males tend to be larger than females, which means, for example, that males can consume more alcohol before causing harm to themselves.

But our bodies are different in other ways too. In fact, as we are about to see, sex determines in large part not just the content of our gut microbiome but also how our bodies will react to possible solutions to issues we have with that same gut microbiome.

Which means quite a lot! Food, drugs, exercise, body mass—all of these have different effects on men than they do on women. So, we will need to get down to the finer details here. Sift through the information we can find. And figure out how, as men or as women, we can understand the effects we have on our gut microbiome and what effect our gut microbiome has on us.

Let's dig into that research then and see what we can't find out.

Animal Studies

So far, animal studies prove that there is a difference in the gut microbial content between male and female animals, specifically in mice. The paper I am using here for reference lists a whole bunch of individual bacteria that are found in higher quantities in female mice, but this is not the kind of book where that specific information is relevant. So, rest assured, at least for now, that there are higher concentrations of certain bacteria in non-obese diabetic female mice than in non-obese diabetic males (Kim *et al.*, 2020).

Now, there have been some studies that appear to suggest little or no difference, but the amount of "noise" in those studies makes such a conclusion difficult. By "noise" here, we mean that diet, age, and genetic background were not sufficiently accounted for.

In studies where the amount of noise has been reduced or accounted for, some interesting findings have occurred. For example, male mice had a lower diversity of gut microbes, but additionally, sex appeared to influence how genes related to immune responses expressed themselves. Considering what we have said already about how our gut microbiome influences our immune responses, this should not be surprising. And yet, it is interesting!

But how diverse the microbiomes are, and maybe whether or not they are diverse at all, might also come down to genotypes. This seemed to be true when inbred strains of mice were studied, which appeared to limit the degree to which sex impacted the diversity of gut microbes.

And yet, even if genotype is the primary cause of whether or not sex influences gut microbe diversity, there are nonetheless cases where sex is a determining factor, i.e., in cases where inbreeding has not occurred.

"Sure," you might be saying. "In mice! But what about human beings?"

Well, are you ever in luck? It's time we turned to...

Human Studies

Without getting into the specifics quite yet, we should start by saying that, as with most things scientific, there do seem to be conflicting reports regarding the influence of sex on the microbiome. This is significant enough that some studies, including one that focused on 91 (i.e., a small number of) northern Europeans, found no evidence that sex impacted microbiome diversity. Meanwhile, another study, which focused on people from many of those same northern countries, found that there was a sex-based difference in colonic microbiota (Kim *et al.*, 2020).

And this is not just limited to these two studies, either. There are maybe a dozen of them where one might say males have a greater abundance of some type of bacteria, and another says this is total bunk. Another says that there is a sex-based difference only in people with certain types of infections, and another says, in fact, that it is only females who have a greater abundance of one type of bacteria.

Reading these studies over, one is faced with a dizzying array of possibilities, where the answer to the question always seems out of reach, if not unreachable.

Thus are the frustrations of science.

But we came here for answers. So, what is the truth here? And where should we be looking to find out?

How about...

Sex Hormones

This is an excellent place to start. The signals here that there is a difference in gut composition between the sexes are strong. So, if we are going to start pulling apart the threads to get to the bottom of this, how sex hormones impact our gut composition appears to lead us to a solution.

Given the topic, however, there is going to be some biochemistry ahead. Hopefully, you have the same enthusiasm for this topic as I do because biochemistry objectively rules. If not, hey, maybe I can convince you!

Either way, we are going to keep this light. And see if this is not the path that leads us up to the light.

Interesting fact right off the hop: Sex differences in gut microbiota do not appear until puberty (Kim *et al.*, 2020). So immediately, the question of whether or not sex hormones affect the microbiome appears to have some level of support, barring some unseen influence.

This gets even more interesting when we look at post-pubertal mice. The gut microbiota of female mice, as it turns out, does not change significantly after puberty. However, there is a not insignificant change in the guts of male mice, meaning male sex hormones (i.e., testosterone) might play a role in altering microbiota compositions.

Furthermore, castrated males had roughly the same microbiota composition as female mice. And when castrated males were treated with testosterone, they developed a microbiota composition that more closely resembled that of their non-castrated counterparts. This is as good a time as any to mention that, yes, I am aware of how strange and dark scientific experimentation can be. But I did not run these experiments! I merely report on them.

Okay, so where are we now? So far, it appears as though the presence of testosterone alters the composition of an individual's microbiome by making it more diverse, which accounts for the sex differences in the gut microbiota of male and female mice after the onset of puberty.

But what about estrogen? Well, several studies also link estrogen production to the microbiome. Particularly, female mice who have their ovaries removed tend to develop dysbiosis. But interestingly, the influence between the microbiome and estrogen appears to run both ways. The reason for this requires a lot of biochemistry, which, frankly, is beyond the scope of this work. But suffice it to say that estrogen seems to keep the microbiome stable, while the microbiome appears to keep estrogen levels stable. Each is tied to the other, and alterations in one create alterations in the other.

To conclude as well as we can here, estrogen and testosterone each appear to influence the gut microbiome in different ways. Considering males typically have more testosterone, while females typically have more estrogen, this means the content *and* behavior of our gut microbiomes are going to differ between males and females.

Again, this is to be taken as "typically" and not "universally." But what all of this suggests is that alterations in the microbiome are going to affect males and females differently. If that proves to be true, then we need to be cautious of how one type of behavior, or diet, may affect one or the other sex.

With that in mind, maybe we should dig a little deeper into...

Diet

Of all the things that modulate gut microbiota composition, diet is maybe the most potent. The fact that it is sex-dependent can also be found across a wide variety of vertebrates. This includes our usual laboratory friends, the mice, but also fish and, yes, humans (Kim *et al.*, 2020).

Fancy talk, I know. Basically, of all the things that are going to alter your microbiome's makeup, diet is the most likely to do so.

How exactly this does so sex-dependently is not clear, however. The state of research on it is still in its infancy, and so those underlying mechanisms have not been uncovered as of this writing. But that does not mean we do not have some idea *that* there is a sex-dependent difference in how food changes our gut microbiomes. In fact, the research on that seems to be as clear as a bell.

Lucky for us, the reasons why this happens are not as important as the apparent fact that it happens at all. For our purposes, the important thing is that the dietary choices of men affect their guts differently than those of women. This means not only that food choices will create different problems between the sexes, but the solutions to these problems vary between men and women, generally speaking.

We will get into what some of these solutions are later, rest assured. But until that happens, I think it is wise for us to simply make a note here that these solutions will be sex-dependent.

Which is interesting! And that is not all, either. Because, as it turns out, there are also sex differences with regard to...

Drugs

That's right: drugs.

But why do drugs matter? Well, one thing we may have noticed is that a good chunk of these studies we have been referring to comment on the gut microbiota of lab mice. Now, there are many ways in which human beings differ from lab mice, not least of all in that they are two different species. Mice may respond to stimuli in similar ways as humans, but the relationship is not 1:1.

The other thing, though, is that laboratory animals are not exposed to the same things as animals in the wild. Diseases are certainly one factor that can come from, say, accidentally eating rotten fruit, which is not likely to occur in a lab. If rotten fruit is encountered at all, it will have been intentionally fed to the lab animal to record how it responds to it.

But for us as humans, we also intentionally ingest drugs. And we do this for a variety of reasons: Drugs are useful as medicine, of course, but we also take them for recreational purposes and sometimes even in dangerous quantities.

Interestingly, both antibiotic and non-antibiotic drugs appear to affect the gut microbiomes of males and females and may account in part for the differences in composition between the sexes (Kim *et al.*, 2020).

Why is this? Well, men and women tend to take different kinds, and even classes, of drugs for different purposes. Men are more likely to take drugs for heart disease, while women are more likely to take opiates, laxatives, and antibiotics. If any of these drugs affect sex hormones, which many of them do, then that, in turn, also affects the gut microbiota, as we discussed earlier.

And, yes, this means that birth control pills change your gut composition.

But let's get back to why we take these drugs in the first place. The fact that men are more likely to take medication for heart disease suggests that men are more susceptible to that problem to begin with. The fact that women are more likely to take antibiotics might suggest that women are more susceptible to bacterial infections.

What is the difference, then, in how the sexes get sick, and what does our gut microbiota have to do with that?

Disease

The fact that the sexes develop different diseases, and that the same disease may present differently between them is now well known. However, why exactly this happens is still a bit of a gray area, although differences in microbiota are a likely culprit (Kim *et al.*, 2020).

Let's take IBS, or irritable bowel syndrome, as a starting point. Women are twice as likely as men to be afflicted with this ailment, which makes it a representative example. Women who have suffered from infectious colitis are at a higher risk of developing IBS than males who have also had colitis, which suggests that, perhaps, the gut microbiome might play some kind of role in setting the stage for irritable bowel syndrome.

Now, one thing that is worth taking note of is that sex hormones are expressed on most immune cells, which in turn influences the sex differences in immune responses. Cool, right? But because the gut microbiota influences the immune cells too, this means that sex hormones and the microbiota are both responsible for immune responses and considering that the types of microbes in male and female bodies differ between the sexes, sex differences in immune responses are effectively coming from two different sides.

In short, male and female bodies respond to disease in different ways due to hormonal and microbial influences on the immune system. Which diseases we are more likely to become infected with is due in part to this immune response, but also *how* we get sick is affected by this.

Consider, for your approval, the Man Cold. When women get a cold, they plow through it terminator-like, rarely affected enough to even have to lie down.

When men get a cold, however, they seem to approach a state resembling death. They require more sleep and complain more... Many of them even suggest that they might be dying.

But why is this? I am speculating here, but considering these sex-specific influences on our immune systems, is it possible that testosterone and the gut microbiota composition play a role in how the disease is expressed differently in men?

Hey, who knows? But it might be worth thinking about.

***

Which leaves us where?

Okay, sex differences are real. We are a sexually dimorphic species, and this is expressed in all kinds of ways. Since we are interested in gut health, we have covered how male and female gut microbiota are influenced, each in their own way, by everything from diet to drugs. We also covered how sex differences in the gut microbiota influence what we get sick with and how we get sick when we do.

But what's the purpose of all this? How does it help us get to where we need to be?

Caring for our gut health as men is different from caring for our gut health as women. Alterations in gut microbiota are going to be expressed differently, which means we will have different problems, and those problems will require sex-specific solutions.

So, on top of being interesting in its own right—which it is, damn you—it is also practical. So, I dunno. You're welcome.

But this is only the beginning! Because up next, we are going to go in for the deep dive. We are going to get into *how* women are affected by gut health, especially how hormonal fluctuations impact it, and what sorts of nutritional strategies we might develop to help with these problems.

It is nothing if not an interesting topic. So, let's quit dallying and get to it.

Chapter 4:
Women and Gut Health

A concept we encounter a lot when reading about gut health is the notion of a "second brain." Why is this? Well, we have already discussed how the gut produces neurotransmitters like serotonin and what effect it has on the immune system. These are jobs traditionally done by the brain, and yet, here is the gut performing those exact same functions.

To the same degree, though? Well, not exactly. Nonetheless, the idea of a second brain is a useful one. It lets us know just how important it is to take care of our gut health—the things we would not do to our brain; in other words, we should not do to our guts either.

For women, this becomes more pronounced. Women's bodies have greater levels of hormonal fluctuation, for example, which means that not taking care of this second brain will impact their mental health to a greater degree. But poor gut health will also impact skin quality, energy levels, and, yes, periods.

This is a lot of ground to cover, though. So, where should we get started?

Tummy Troubles

We've all been there. We have felt bloated and nauseous, and we have had heartburn. These sorts of problems are a part of everyday life, and honestly, for women, many of these problems wind up going unaddressed.

Why is this? Well, who knows? But the fact of the matter is that while everybody, men included, has tummy problems, they can mean different things for women. Not addressing them, therefore, can be quite a mistake.

But we are getting ahead of ourselves.

An interesting fact about women's digestive systems: Women are more likely to be "supertasters" than men (Reddy, 2022). What does this mean? It means that women are better able to taste bitter and sweaty flavors at a much stronger level than men. And actually, the female GI tract is way more sensitive in all kinds of areas.

For example, heartburn—female esophagi squeeze shut with more force than the male versions, which means there is less of a chance of damage resulting from the stomach acids. But, since women are more sensitive to irritants, they will feel heartburn more strongly than men do. So, a bit of a quid pro quo.

We have already discussed how women are more susceptible to irritable bowel syndrome. But see, it comes from that same sensitivity to irritants. Alas, IBS comes with a whole host of nasty symptoms, which means this sensitivity to irritants is turning out to be a little more quid than pro, if you know what I mean.

And here is another one: Women's digestive systems empty with less frequency than men's digestive systems. This might be, in fact, why women are more likely to experience symptoms of nausea, even when there is not an obvious external cause.

Also, women's intestines are 10cm longer than men. This is an interesting fact, even if I do not understand the evolutionary purpose of such a thing. And even with that extra length of the intestine, all these digestive organs have to share space with the reproductive ones. So, a woman's stomach is much more crowded than a man's.

All this to say that when something has gone awry in a woman's digestive tract, it is probably because of an innate, increased sensitivity to irritants in that system. But it could also be because of other things that are specific to the female digestive system.

Beyond the digestive tract, however, there is also the issue of hormones. And specifically, how those hormones affect, and are affected by, gut health.

So, let's wade into these waters now and see what we can't find out.

Hormones

First off, it's time for a new word: "estrobolome."

Crazy word, right? The estrobolome is the collection of gut bacteria that modulate and metabolize the body's estrogen, or the "bridge between gut health and hormones" (The Nutrition Professionals, 2022).

How this happens is a little complicated. But in simple terms, estrogen is primarily broken down in the liver. Once this happens, it is then circulated via bile and comes into contact with gut bacteria. These microbes then synthesize an enzyme that allows estrogen to be reabsorbed into the body, basically converting inactive estrogen into active estrogen.

When the balance is thrown off, and dysbiosis occurs, the body can wind up with either too much or too little estrogen (also known as "dominance" or "deficiency"). The common symptoms of dysbiosis we have discussed earlier, but for the sake of refreshing our memories, they include: upset stomach, constipation, diarrhea, bloating, gas, fatigue, and bad breath. In other words, dysbiosis is not a desirable state to be in.

But what about when this dysbiosis also causes estrogen dominance or deficiency? What happens then?

As it turns out, there are a whole host of other horrible symptoms. You can wind up with: cramps, bloating, heavy periods, irritability, and PMS-related symptoms.

And if you wind up with estrogen dominance specifically, well, that ain't no cakewalk either. The symptoms differ between men and women, but in women they include: bloating, decreased sex drive, irregular periods, headaches, weight gain, hair loss, and fatigue.

In men, the symptoms are different. But since this helps corroborate my claims that the bodies of men and women are different enough to warrant different methods of care, I am going to list those also.

So, here are the symptoms of estrogen dominance in men: infertility, gynecomastia (colloquially known as "man boobs"), and erectile dysfunction.

Okay, with that out of the way, what does it all mean?

Gut health and hormone production are intimately linked to one another. Since hormone production and absorption, the making of inactive estrogen, say, into active estrogen, as well as the metabolizing of the same, are dependent on good gut health, we need to take care of our guts; otherwise, we wind up with one or more of those awful symptoms listed above.

For women, the issue of how estrogen is affected by gut health is especially important. Because while men have estrogen, it is more prevalent in women, and imbalances are the cause of a whole host of problems, it would be wiser to avoid them.

The question then is, *what exactly can women do to prevent this from happening?*

Because, yes, I have spent a lot of time talking about what happens when we let our gut health go by the wayside. I think/hope you are adequately informed about the importance of gut health by now—at least enough that I can get into some nutritional strategies.

If not, well, you can't say I didn't try. Here are some nutritional strategies women can adopt to keep their guts healthy:

Nutrition for Women

Alright, ladies. It is time to get into the weeds here.

What sorts of things can we do to make sure our guts remain healthy enough that hormonal problems do not result from our negligence?

Well, considering we are talking about our digestive systems, the first thing we should be thinking about is food. What we eat has, as you can imagine, an enormous impact on our gut health. So, for this section, I would like to run over the kinds of foods we should be eating, i.e., which ones have a specific, positive effect on our gut microbiome.

First, there are the ever-handy probiotics. These are foods that contain the kinds of bacteria that makes our guts healthy (Solgar, 2023).

Of these, yogurt is probably the most well-known for having this property. But if and when you buy some, make sure it has active or live cultures—not all yogurt is created equal. Some yogurts are healthier than others, so check your labels before making your purchase.

Sauerkraut is another probiotic, although its popularity, as I have noticed, is anything but consistent across populations. Some people really hate the stuff!

Funny story: One time, when I had first moved out on my own, I bought a can of sauerkraut and opened it to put on some burgers. But seeing as I was new to being on my own, I figured topping off the can with plastic wrap and elastic would be sufficient for when I put it back in the fridge.

What I did not realize was that the smell of the sauerkraut would leak into everything in the fridge. And with this, the taste of sauerkraut was in everything. And I mean *everything*. The apples tasted like sauerkraut. Even the milk did, which is about as gross a combination as I can imagine.

I spent over an hour trying everything in the fridge to see what survived. And, of course, nothing did. The sauerkraut destroyed all my food, and I had to throw everything out and start again.

In other words, it was a while before I could eat sauerkraut again. So, I get it; I understand why some people do not like it. But even after all that, I eventually came around to it again. And now I use it all the time!

Kimchi is another probiotic that is super popular. You can pretty well put this in any dish and make it a gazillion times better. Burritos, pasta, whatever—just huck some kimchi in there, and you are having a party.

And lastly, pickles are a probiotic! And who the heck doesn't like pickles?

Now, some of you might be asking, "What about kombucha? I heard that's good for your gut health."

And you would be right! Kombucha is good for your gut. And not only that, it has antioxidants too, which should always be a part of your diet. So yeah, go nuts with kombucha. It's great.

Fiber, too, is an important part of gut health. Fiber is non-digestible matter, which helps keep your stool soft, and therefore, helps keep things moving down there, if you know what I mean.

So, which foods are high in fiber?

Well, you cannot really go wrong with beans. Specifically, garbanzo, kidney, and pinto beans are among those with the highest fiber content. Plus, they taste good, and you can put them in everything from salads to burritos. (In case you can't tell, I am going through a burrito phase.)

Broccoli is another one that is high in fiber. For some reason, people are either moderately for or passionately against this vegetable. I do not understand this. Broccoli is awesome. Just putting it on rice with a bit of vinegar is great for a snack, so long as the rice is brown.

Fruits, in general, are great for fiber, but berries specifically have this property. Strawberries, blackberries, blueberries... And honestly, who the heck doesn't like fruit? I have only known a couple of people who have expressed ambivalence about fruit, and I refuse to trust their judgment in any capacity after that. Fruit is fantastic. And you cannot possibly eat too much of it, no matter what those keto people tell you.

Lastly, the avocado. This is a tricky one because it is fattier than other fruits and vegetables. But it is really good for you. They have tons of B vitamins and C vitamins. And, yes, fiber. Some people are iffy on the avocado, but not me. I love these things.

So much for what you should be eating. What about the things you should stay away from? What kinds of foods are bad for women's gut health—or gut health in general?

Bad Foods: Stay Away!

Alright, look, nobody likes to be told what to do. Right? It is way more inviting to say, "Check out all these things we *can* do! They make us healthy, and they make us feel better! Do these things *all you want!*"

But unfortunately, life does not come without its share of dos and don'ts. When it comes to food, though, there is a caveat that comes with listing foods we should stay away from. Because obsessing over which foods we should not eat is only going to make us more unhealthy, as ironic as that might seem.

The reason? Well, a good chunk of that is mental. Obsessing over food restrictions is likely to cause an eating disorder if it is not already a symptom of an existing one. But the other thing is that inevitably, we will eat food that is not 100% good for us. And if we have already been focusing on never eating unhealthy food, we run the risk of developing sunk cost syndrome— namely, that we think, "Well, I obviously can't keep the promises I make. So, I might as well just pull the chute and eat as much junk as I want."

This is how yo-yo dieting starts. And yo-yo dieting is super unhealthy. So how do we get around this?

We need to have realistic expectations. We need to remember that we will sometimes eat food that is not 100% good for us, and that is totally okay. So long as we eat mostly healthy most of the time, we are going to be in a really good place.

With that in mind, the foods we are about to discuss here are not to be taken as though I am referring to poison. They are not dangerous in sensible quantities, and it is okay to occasionally indulge in them.

That being said, overindulgence in these foods is not going to be good for the ol' gut health. So, without further ado, here are the foods that should be sensibly avoided if we are going to take the central thesis of this book seriously.

First of all, there are the artificial sweeteners. This is a tough one to list here because it has become a popular alternative to sugar. And honestly, the white, granulated sugar we throw into our food and drinks is really, really not good for us.

But artificial sweeteners really do wretched things to our gut health. These include common ones like sucralose, saccharin, and aspartame. As an alternative, you might see if you can handle black coffee or try natural sweeteners like honey.

The next item on the list is processed foods. Really, this should be no surprise. Processed foods are terrible for us. All the time, we hear about how some of them might be carcinogenic, how they put our hearts through the wringer... But to that list, we can add that they are super bad for our guts as well.

But why is this? Well, processed foods tend to be low in fiber and high in sugar. These, coupled with the artificial preservatives, do not provide adequate environments for healthy bacteria to grow. And so, if we needed any further reasons to limit our intake of processed foods, they can help cause the problems with gut microbiome composition we have been discussing throughout this book.

Next up is fried food.

Damn, but this is a hard one, right? Who the heck doesn't like fried food? So many American staples are fried. Some places even have grand traditions of fried foods, including New England fried calamari and cheese curds throughout the Midwest.

Alas, fried foods are really unhealthy. And some of this we know already! Or, at least, we would if we were paying attention, even slightly. This is the information we are inundated with regularly: How fried food clogs your arteries, how it makes you obese, and therefore causes all kinds of health problems—including cancer.

But the grease is not good for your gut health either. Think about what happens to your stomach when you eat too much of it in the first place. I would rather not go into details, but I think we all know what I am talking about.

Imagine doing that to your stomach regularly over long periods of time. Your gut health is not going to be in working order. It is going to be out of whack.

Which means, unfortunately, that our intake of fried foods needs to be limited. Again, not eliminated, because that is not sensible. But limited.

And lastly, the hardest one of all: alcohol.

Culturally, there are few more ubiquitous elements in a social setting. Alcohol is connected to all sorts of things: It is part of having a night out, and it is part of relaxing. It is one of the first things that comes to mind when we think of going on a vacation or meeting up with an old friend.

It is even tied to social class. Fancy dinners are treated to wine, and pub crawls are filled with beer. Scotch is for men in suits, and whiskey is for men in overalls.

And it has been around forever, too. Wine was an important part of early Western culture, both in Greece and Rome. It is considered sacramental in Christianity. And supposedly, one of the earliest pieces of writing we have is a beer recipe from ancient Babylon.

Which is why, in many ways, it is so unfortunate that alcohol is so dangerous. It is a cause of missed days at work due to hangovers, car accidents because of drunk driving... Alcoholism destroys families and ruins lives. It is a contributing factor to homelessness and spousal abuse.

And on top of all that, it is wickedly bad for our gut health.

Much like with fried food, this is an easy connection to make. Think of what your stomach feels like the day after drinking. Think of the nausea, the vomiting—heck, even think of the vomiting *while still drunk*.

Have you ever been near a drunk person's breath? It smells awful. There is every indication that alcohol does terrible things to our gut health. And if that is what we are concerned with here... ?

But, again, we need to be realistic. As we just said, alcohol is an integral part of our social lives. And while many of us do not drink at all, me included, it is often at the risk of social isolation. An effort has to be made to be a sober person during a night out.

So yes, eliminating alcohol is not an option for some people. Which is totally cool. But knowledge is power, and we should know that when we do indulge in it, it is playing havoc with our guts. And when that happens, health problems can arise.

***

So yes, ladies, there are some unique, sex-specific challenges ahead when considering gut health. Women's bodies endure hormonal fluctuations in ways that men's bodies do not, and they have a much more sensitive digestive system. For this reason, irritants in the gut are way more likely to affect women, which means causing more problems more quickly.

Poor gut health can cause estrogen dominance or deficiency, which comes with a whole host of undesirable symptoms. Gut health and estrogen stability are uniquely tied together, which means women have an entire area of health to worry about that men do not.

Luckily, proper nutrition, both by eating good foods and avoiding bad ones, can be a solution to this problem. Fibrous diets, low in alcohol and fried food consumption, are a good place to start.

But that can't be all, can it? Is it really just as simple as monitoring our food intake? Is it really just a matter of not eating junk or drinking too much?

Not in your life! In fact, there is a super cool method for keeping our guts healthy that I would like to introduce you to.

So, keep on reading and learn the secrets of the *gut cleanse!*

Chapter 5:
Balancing the Gut—the Gut Cleanse

We have all known someone who has gone on a cleanse by now, have we not? For me, the first time I heard of it was in high school. I was taking an environmental science course, which was less heavy on the science part but still interesting.

Anyway, my teacher was always going on a cleanse, it seemed. He would try a new one every few weeks or so, such as ones where he could only drink juice or ones where he would flood his body with vitamins. He swears by them, and I developed an immediate interest in trying it out for myself.

So, before we get started, we should define what exactly we are talking about here.

"Gut cleanse," "digestive cleanse," "colon cleanse"—these are all more or less the same things. What they refer to is a method by which accumulations of feces are removed from the digestive system.

I know, gross. The idea, though, is that these accumulations are bad things, and removing them is a good thing. Doing so requires what are basically simple procedures, some of them good, some of them ineffective.

The thing is, there are a lot of ins and outs and a lot of what-have-yous. And while a single chapter in one book is not going to cover every single thing you could possibly want to know about doing a cleanse, I hope that what I have put in here at least sets you on the right path.

So, with that in mind, let's start with the obvious question:

Why Should We Do a Cleanse?

Alright, let's get the big thing out of the way: The research on the effectiveness of cleanses is scant at best. There are a lot of questions that have not been answered, which has not stopped some people from making all kinds of outlandish claims about the benefits of this practice (White, 2023).

That being said, there are many people who claim that a colon cleanse, in particular, comes with a whole host of benefits. Those people tend to really swear by them, which is either a good or a bad thing, depending on how you see colon cleanses to begin with.

What we can say for sure is that there are times when doing a colon cleanse is important. To relieve constipation is an obvious one, but cleansing before a colonoscopy is sometimes advisable.

Under circumstances like these, the preferred method seems to be what is known as "colon hydrotherapy." This is, in essence, an enema—water is used to wash out, or flush out, all the, uh, crap that is inside you. That this relieves constipation is obvious, but how it impacts a colonoscopy should be clear too: There are no visual impediments, as it were, to seeing and inspecting the colon.

But if we were to do this in a non-medical setting, is this the method we should use? Well...

Methods for Cleaning Your Digestive System

First off, there are a whole bunch of instruments you can get in stores and online that are marketed as performing colon cleanses. To go through all of them here would take way too long, and so I am not going to use this section to review individual products and claims. The things I am interested in are the at-home, "diet and exercise" ways we can flush our digestive systems out, and so that is what I am going to focus on.

Starting off with the most accessible one: Drinking plenty of water (White, 2023).

That is right, *water*. Staying hydrated is a great way to regulate your digestive system. Lukewarm water is great for this in particular, but you can also eat lots of water-rich foods, like fruits and vegetables, for similar effects.

And of course, those fruits and vegetables include such awesome things as watermelon, celery, and tomatoes. Who doesn't like those?

It is also possible to do one using salt water. This is known as a "saltwater flush" and is really only used for constipation. But there are people, it seems, who swear that by drinking lukewarm salt water, they undergo a significant cleansing of their bowels.

If you do decide to go this route, you should, of course, talk to your doctor first. But if you get the okay, what you can do is mix a couple of teaspoons of salt (even Himalayan salt, if you are into that sort of thing) and drink it first thing in the morning on an empty stomach.

This should make you go to the bathroom within minutes. In fact, you will likely need to do this multiple times. Do this in the morning and at night, and *bam*, you will have been cleansed.

If drinking salt water does not sound good to you, though, you can also get on the fiber. Which, really, you should do anyway. Fiber is super good for you.

Fiber bulks out whatever you eat so that it passes through your colon with greater ease. Low-fiber diets have all kinds of horrible side effects, from constipation to chronic bouts of diarrhea, and so it follows that high-fiber diets will likely not result in either of those things.

Seriously, fiber is super good for you. Make sure you get lots of it.

There is also the ever-popular juice cleanse, which can also involve using smoothies. However, there is an even greater dearth of evidence that these work than for cleanses as a whole. In fact, the so-called Master's Diet, which promotes heavy amounts of juice and broth to both lose weight and "detoxify" the body, really just makes you starve.

The other thing too, is that juice has less fiber than unjuiced fruit. Fruit is insanely good for you, and eating lots of it helps promote weight loss on its own. So why not just eat boatloads of fruit instead of doing a juice cleanse?

Anyway, that is my two cents.

In addition to fiber, you can also throw in some resistant starches. These starches are found in potatoes, rice, and green bananas. They act in a similar way to fiber, which means, for us colon people, that they can help with the ol' cleanse in an appropriately similar way.

The thing is, some people are on low-carb diets, and so this will not be an option for them. *Or so you would think!*

You can totally eat green bananas or lentils on a low-carb diet and get these resistant starches at the same time. So, if that is where you are at, I would recommend that route.

And moving on, we have the probiotics. We already went through a bunch of these (yogurt, kimchi), so I will not go into a super amount of detail here. But for gut cleanses, these can be fantastic.

In particular, people seem really taken in by apple cider vinegar. While there are very few animal-based studies on its effectiveness, there are all kinds of claims circulating about how it fights off bad bacteria, infections, etc. A whole bunch of things.

For this reason, people like to drink it in purified water, along with, perhaps, a bit of honey to help it go down more smoothly. The thinking is that by having it travel through your system, it will neutralize the toxins and bad bacteria, thereby making you healthier.

Again, the jury is out on this one. But at the very least, it looks like it can't *hurt*. Which is not nothing!

And finally, we have the herbal teas.

As it turns out, there are such things as laxative herbal teas. These include psyllium, aloe vera, marshmallow root, and slippery elm. Given, however, that these are laxatives, it is possible to use them too much. You can dilute yourself into poor health.

But if used sparingly?

Well, I wish I could tell you they for sure worked. But, again, the jury is out on this one. There are claims too, about how things like cayenne pepper neutralize bad bacteria, but there really is not that much information on this.

As usual, it is best that you talk to your doctor first. They can give you a better idea than I can about whether or not herbal laxative teas are a healthy method for you to adopt should you decide to embark on a cleanse.

But even if this is not the right method for you, there are still, as we have seen, a boatload of other methods available to get the cleanse going. And as usual, eating tons of fruit and drinking lots of water is the best thing for you: It will keep you regular and healthy, make sure things are moving down there, and are not prone to side effects.

Which reminds me...

Side Effects

Yeah, this is something we have to get into for a little bit.

See, any of these cleanses other than fruit and water come with side effects. Which does not mean they do not work. But if you do decide to try a cleanse, you will want to come in knowing what to expect and what to do if you encounter any of these hurdles I am about to go through.

In the worst-case scenario, it is possible that you might develop one of these symptoms:

Inflammation of the colon or bowels

Electrolyte imbalances

Dehydration

Infection

If any of these things happen to you, you should contact your doctor immediately. These are life-threatening, any one of them in particular, since they can induce not just digestive failure but heart failure. Bowel perforation is also a possibility, which can lead to sepsis.

If you decide to go the enema route, this is not going to cause you any problems if it is only done occasionally. The risk that doing one often poses is that you can wind up chronically constipated and become dependent on them. And you can damage your bowels.

With herbal teas, some herbs do not interact well with medication. Antidepressants, for example, should not be taken in combination with St. John's Wort. So, keep that in mind.

As far as what we should do if and when we encounter these symptoms, well, that is clear: For the severe ones, call a doctor. For the less severe ones, we should think about whether or not this type of cleansing is really the right choice for us.

I can't overstate enough how drinking tons of water and getting lots of fiber does not result in these types of symptoms. But, of course, many of these might sound like attractive options to you, and so really, just keep an eye on your body, know if and when something has gone wrong, and drink tons of water anyway. Especially if you are using a laxative tea, dehydration can result quite quickly. Consider drinking more water than you normally do to make up for what you are losing.

Under normal circumstances, that would be where I close things out. What more is there to talk about now that we have gone through the possible methods, the possible side effects, and what the recommendations are for mitigating the risks and boosting the benefits?

Alas, there is one more method that we need to talk about. It is a popular one that often finds its way into the news as an object of ridicule. And since some of you might be interested in this, I have decided to include it here, giving it its own space so it can be dealt with appropriately.

Of course, I am talking about...

The Coffee Enema

If we do not know what this is, do not worry; the name really gives itself away. Effectively, a person inserts brewed and caffeinated coffee into their colon as an enema instead of the usual, regular-ass water (McDermott, 2017).

Interesting fact about them: They originated in Germany as a possible cancer treatment. Obviously, that did not pan out, but that did not stop the coffee enema from making its way into our collective consciousness.

The man who first popularized it was a fellow named Max Gerson. He was a popularizer of various folk remedies, which are collectively known as "Gerson therapy." His recommendations included all sorts of ways of removing so-called toxins from the body, particularly through the use of an organic, plant-based diet, raw juices, and, yes, the coffee enema.

Now, in case you can't tell by my tone, I am nothing if not skeptical of this treatment. Nonetheless, I would like to give it its due, even if I only do so briefly. And so here I am going to run through the supposed benefits of this procedure and then break down what the research says about it.

So, here we go:

The Alleged Benefits of the Coffee Enema

Coffee is a bit of a laxative when consumed orally, so imagine what it does when consumed rectally. Multiple bowel movements are often reported as an immediate effect, which, for some people, might be a good thing.

Another sure thing users get from it is a boost of energy. Caffeine is clearly the culprit here. By bypassing the usual digestive route, you get a higher concentration of the drug in much the same way that rectal suppositories work. Drug addicts too will partake of what they call "booty bumping," where they shove heroin or cocaine into their rectum, usually after all other methods of consumption have been destroyed by drug use.

Which is not to say that coffee enemas have anything in common with booty bumping other than the obvious. I am only saying that as a method of delivery, your ass is totally able to absorb drugs in high concentrations, which will, yes, allow you to feel their effects to a greater degree.

Beyond this, supporters also claim that the coffee enema can boost your immune system, stop yeast overgrowth, remove parasites, rid your digestive system of heavy metals, treat depression, and, maybe most importantly of all, treat cancer.

But how much of this is true? What does the research say?

The Research

Unfortunately—or fortunately, depending on your perspective—no research has been done to test whether or not the coffee enema is capable of doing any of the things its supporters claim it can do. All of these claims are anecdotal and have never been tested in a clinical trial.

For this reason, there are not even medical guidelines detailing who should or should not partake of them. But there is some evidence of harmful side effects, which should, I will argue, dissuade people from attempting this type of cleanse.

To begin with, the medical literature recognizes three deaths that have occurred as a result of coffee enemas. Two of these were due to an electrolyte imbalance, and one of them may have been because of a bacterial infection.

A woman in Korea also suffered inflammation of the colon as a result of the procedure, which is not a comfortable experience.

But as if that were not enough, consider these other possible side effects:

Since this is brewed coffee we are talking about, some people have burned their rectums as a result of using *hot coffee* instead of doing the sensible thing and waiting for it to cool down first. The caffeine overload can also lead to nausea, vomiting, cramping, and bloating.

The equipment, too, can cause problems. If you come in too strong and the equipment is sturdy enough, you can wind up with bowel perforation. And if it is not adequately sanitized? God help you.

The other thing is that most places charge an arm and a leg for one of these things. So, on top of there being no recognized medical benefit, and with all these side effects waiting around the corner, it is super expensive.

Should you get one, then? No. I mean, that is just me. But I would not recommend these things. There are a gazillion better ways than this to go through a cleanse, none of which come with the same risk level.

Do yourself a favor, then. Skip the coffee enema.

***

So, let's go over the points we made here one more time.

Cleanses are super popular. Lots of people swear by them, and plenty of people are interested in them for a variety of reasons. There is very little medical research to suggest that they work, but there is lots of anecdotal evidence that there might be some benefits.

Of the methods we went over, some of them were sensible, others not so much. Sticking with tons of water and fiber is always going to be your best ticket, but if you are interested in trying some other things, I hope this list was helpful.

And no matter what you think you might get out of it, stay away from the coffee enema.

That about sums that up, folks. So where are we now?

Well, the topic of mental health has been referenced a few times. Certainly, it is a big one and certainly something we should be concerned about.

We know that gut health and mental health are connected. But how and to what degree? What sorts of problems might we encounter with regard to our mental health when undertaking a journey to greater gut health?

Let's find out.

Chapter 6:
Mental Health and the Gut

In some ways, mental health is one of the more pressing issues of our time. Its effects are everywhere, from the anxiety epidemic in teenagers to the homelessness crisis in virtually every major city in North America—most of which are made up of people with untreated mental health disorders.

How we treat it and how we even *talk* about it are constant sources of discussion. We have a whole industry built around this—and I mean that in a good way. We have everything from therapists to pharmaceutical interventions, exercise programs, etc.

So, as we go forward in this chapter, it should be noted that none of what is in here is intended to replace any of that. Mental health is complicated and, frankly, not very well understood, even after all this time. Much of why we have episodes of poor mental health, and especially how that happens, is unknown to us.

Nonetheless, there does appear to be a connection between our gut health and our mental health. And so here, we are going to explore the gut-brain axis, the vagus nerve, and a whole bunch of other cool things in order to do our best to get to the bottom of this phenomenon.

So, with that, let's start with the obvious.

How Are the Gut and Brain Connected?

Okay, so the common term that is used to describe this connection is one we have already covered in an earlier chapter: The "gut-brain axis" (Robertson, 2023). This is a network of communication that exists between the two systems. This connection is both physical and biochemical, and in a whole bunch of different ways.

We have already covered a bit about the number of neurons in your brain as well as the number of neurons in your gut. But among all of these, the vagus nerve is the largest one connecting the two systems; in fact, it sends signals in both directions.

Want an example? Well, don't mind if I do.

In animal studies, when the vagus nerve is inhibited by stress, it causes gastrointestinal problems. People with IBS and Crohn's disease, too, have been shown to have reduced function in the vagus nerve.

A study in mice also found that probiotics reduced the amount of stress hormone in their blood, *unless the vagus nerve was severed*. If this were done, the probiotics would have had no effect on stress whatsoever.

This gives us good reason to think that this gut-brain axis is more than just theoretical and that, via the vagus nerve, it might be possible to reduce the effect of stress on our bodies through changes in our diet.

In Chapter 1, we also addressed how the gut is a source of the precursors to our neurotransmitters, including serotonin and GABA. So, rest assured, we are not going to reiterate any of that here. We also know how the gut is connected to the immune system, but what we didn't cover is that through our immune systems, our guts being out of order can lead to inflammation.

Why is this? Well, when your immune system is "switched on" for too long, this leads to inflammation. And why this is important for us is that depression and schizophrenia, as well as Alzheimer's, might be connected to chronic inflammation.

Mental Health and Inflammation

First of all, we are going to address the link between inflammation and depression.

This is a bit of a tricky one. There is a tendency, I think, amongst some reporters to look at some findings around inflammation and depression and say, "Oh, look: Depression is an inflammatory disorder!"

Alas, this is false. Depression is not an inflammatory disorder. Furthermore, not all inflammatory disorders can lead to depression, and not all people with depression have signs of inflammation (Miller, 2018). So, the connection between these two things is way more nuanced than you are likely to find in your average news article.

The thing too, is that while inflammation is found in a certain (albeit unknown) percentage of the population with depression, it is also found in people with anxiety disorders, schizophrenia, and others. So, it is not that inflammation causes one or the other psychiatric disorder; rather, it is what we would call "transdiagnostic," or found across multiple different but connected diagnoses.

One thing that can be said positively is that inflammation seems to play a role in whether or not patients respond to treatment. There is, for example, a whole class of treatment-resistant depression in which the patient does not respond to medication. But with inflammation being targeted as the culprit behind this, a therapeutic response to this class of disorder might very well be imminent.

And what, pray tell, might be a preferred pathway to dealing with this problem? Well...

Probiotics

By now, we should know what these are, so I am not going to summarize that again here. What we need to know for now is that these wonderful products, since they affect gut health, likely affect brain health as well.

In fact, there is a name for probiotics that affect the brain: "psychobiotics."

One study that sought to test the effects of probiotics on depression, in particular, found that participants with major depressive disorder who had taken larger amounts of probiotics than the other group had far fewer depressive symptoms (Akkasheh *et al.*, 2016).

The symptoms were measured using what is called the Beck Depression Inventory (BDI). This is a test that asks participants to self-report symptoms correlated with depression—how sad they are feeling, for example.

Using the BDI, then, it appeared as though probiotics alleviated the symptoms of depression.

And that is not all. Participants who took probiotics also had observable improvements with regard to insulin, homeostasis, and a whole bunch of other things.

So, do they work? Well, this is only one study. Of course, it seems like they work, and if more studies confirm this, then that is fantastic. We should not get our hopes up, of course, but since gut and mental health are connected, taking care of the gut, for example, by using probiotics, should, logically, help take care of mental health.

But what about the other way? Can taking care of our mental health have a positive effect on our gut health? What sorts of mental health strategies might we adopt to keep our guts healthy and happy?

Mental Health Strategies

First off, we have already discussed how anxiety causes gastrointestinal problems. So, I think the jury is no longer out on whether or not caring for our mental well-being affects our digestive well-being.

But, of course, taking care of our mental health can be a challenge. As we said earlier, there is a whole industry built up around this, and for good reason. Not only is it worth worrying about, but being mentally healthy requires all sorts of different things to be in the right place, from how we think to how we eat, how we exercise, and everything in between.

There are some things we can do on our own, however. And those are the things I would like to get into here.

Staying Connected

There are some lone wolves out there, no doubt. Some people really like being alone; they like the freedom they have to think without having to worry about other people.

I have always been a big reader of horror stories, and the writers of these tales seem to be loners to a greater degree than in other fictional fields. The one that mostly comes to mind, I think, when we think of isolated horror writers is HP Lovecraft.

For those of you who do not know him, he was a New England writer who wrote famously dark stories about cosmic entities destroying the sanity of whoever was unfortunate enough to discover them. His influence is so pervasive that, at this point, it is impossible to discuss the history of horror without mentioning his name. There is a good chance, in fact, that he may be one of the most skilled writers who ever lived.

As a personality, he was famously isolated much of the time. Most of his friends he only knew through correspondence. And he was only married once, and for a brief period. He liked to stay in his hometown of Providence, Rhode Island, reading and writing and, seemingly, doing little else.

But even though there is a kind of mystique around a writer who lives alone and writes stories of sheer horror, he nonetheless *did* have friends. He did not get out a whole lot for most of his life, but he did eventually discover a love of travel.

In other words, the idea of the loner, even in someone who seems to embody it best, is still a myth. It is a fantasy. Consider some of our great fictional loners, from John Rambo to Clint Eastwood's *Man with No Name*. They appeal to the part of us that wants to be free, but they remain fantasies. There is not a person alive, I do not think, who can withstand being completely isolated from other people for too long. Not, that is, without going full-on Travis Bickle.

All this is to say that staying connected to people is an important part of staying healthy. Even if we do not get to see people often, we still have to see them *sometimes*. Even if they drive us absolutely insane, we still have to say hello, even if it is only now and then.

Okay, so we need to be social. But we also need...

Exercise

I know. I am not happy about this either.

I am a fully indoor person. I enjoy reading and writing, and I love music. None of these things require me to get out much. And yet, if I do not exercise? Well, I am not different from anybody else. Not exercising means trouble.

And while we know that not exercising does horrible things to our bodies, it also does horrible things to our brains. Exercise helps relieve anxiety, for one, and can help stave off depressive episodes, as I can attest from personal experience.

Now, some people love exercise. If that's you, great! But some people do not care for exercise at all, and yet they still have to get up and move their bodies or risk the side effects.

The trick here is really just to get into the habit. Which is harder than it sounds, but it is true. Once you start exercising, it is really important to just keep doing it. It becomes a part of your routine, even when you wind up craving it. Your brain, remember, gets addicted to things; being addicted to running is not a bad thing. At least, when compared to the other things we get addicted to.

So as much as it might stink, exercise is the lynchpin, along with diet, when it comes to our health. It is good for us physically and good for us mentally, and since it helps improve our mental well-being, then, by extension, it keeps our guts happy too.

But wait—there's more!

Learning New Skills

Having a sense of accomplishment is key to emotional well-being. Accomplishing things gives our lives meaning. We feel like we are becoming something grand, something better than what we were before.

Do these skills have to be big and grand things, then? No, of course not. Even just learning the basics of a new language or the rudiments of a musical instrument can help bring on these feelings of joy at having *done* something. It can help us feel like we do not have to stagnate and wither away. If you like, it makes us feel like we can take life by the horns.

The thing about a state like depression is that it makes us think that these types of things are not possible. Far more than just being really sad, depression is a genuinely pathological state in which hope, and meaning are drained from reality. What is left is something dark and terrifying, and, it seems, impossible to get out of.

There is some talk that major depression might be the least desirable mental state one can be in. By its nature, it is impossible to suffer (mentally, that is) as much as a person does when depressed. And part of that comes from the fact that meaning and hope are requirements for our well-being.

Our flourishing, then, comes at least in part from becoming the kind of person we would like to be. And that person, for most of us, is one who can grow and adapt. Feeling like we are not at the mercy of forces beyond our control.

Learning new skills reinforces that, I think. It reminds us that even if things get wild, we can adapt. All we have to do to remember this is to do something small to confirm that we are capable of change and, therefore, of survival.

Alright, enough high-minded talk. The conclusion here is that learning new things makes us feel better mentally, and feeling better mentally makes our guts happy and healthy. But taking care of our mental well-being extends to all kinds of other areas of flourishing, so it should not be neglected.

It is just as important as exercise if you ask me. And since you are reading this book, I suppose, in a way, that you are.

Mental Health in America

With all that said, you might be asking: Is this a problem worth worrying about? How many people are affected by mental health anyway?

Boy, am I ever glad you asked? Except not because this topic stinks.

The first thing to take note of is that an overwhelming majority of Americans at least appear to recognize that there is a mental crisis in their home country (McPhillips, 2022). In fact, according to a poll conducted by CNN and the Kaiser Family Foundation, 90% of Americans believe the United States is in a mental health crisis. Which is an enormous number, no matter who you are.

That said, it is important to note that this poll was taken about two and a half years after the onset of the COVID-19 pandemic. And the reason why that timing is important is that the pandemic obviously exacerbated a lot of problems, from mental illness to substance abuse.

That being said, when participants were asked to name the six areas of specific concern with regards to a mental health crisis, the opioid crisis came out on top. And this is not a matter of misperception, either. Drug overdose deaths hit record levels in 2021, and suicides were back to near their peak after two years of declining rates.

And it gets worse. In 2020, mental health-related emergency visits among those aged 12–17 rose by 34%. Half of the adults polled said they have had a mental health emergency with at least one family member. One in five people described their own mental health as either "fair" or "poor."

The statistics go on, of course, but none of them get any prettier. The fact of the matter is that something has slipped into the collective American psyche. Huge numbers of us are ill. Loneliness and isolation remain problems even after the pandemic.

Now, part of the problem, for my money, is that there is this pervasive assumption that problems are monocausal. This is true of mental health as much as it is of anything else. So, you will see people say things like, "The problem is we have a culture of nihilism." Or "The problem is we have machines doing all our work, and that has caused us to live without purpose." Or, yes, "The problem is that we eat nothing but junk."

But the truth is that a lot of different things are creating this problem. Hell, probably every single thing, minus the really wild ones (like the government putting things in our water), probably has at least some truth to it.

So, as I said earlier, there is just no way that promoting gut health can fix the mental health crisis in America.

But can it not at least do *something*? Can it not at least be part of what makes things better?

Maybe we really do need to regain some spiritual center that has been lost in the last, well, few decades at the very least. Maybe we do need to rely less on technology, both for our work and for socializing.

And maybe we need to focus on what we put into our bodies, too. Because maybe this enormous cluster of influences is making our brains sick, each in their own way.

So, as I have said before, and as I will say a thousand times, there is no "insert one solution to solve all problems" device. Everything is more complicated than it initially appears. Everything.

But diet and mental health really do seem to be connected. And given how dire things look in America right now, with that awful opioid crisis only getting worse all the time and self-harm on the rise... Should we not keep an open mind about where parts of our solutions might come from?

Do we not need all the help we can get?

***

Alright. Where are we now?

Mental health and gut health are connected to each other, and each affects the other. Taking care of one, then, helps take care of the other.

By eating well, including taking in probiotics, we can help fend off the effects of inflammation, which might (*might*) help prevent certain mental health disorders, including depression. And by taking care of our mental health, we might be able to keep our guts healthy.

So now that we have talked about the mind, it is time to talk about the body.

We know diet and exercise are important. But in the next chapter, we are going to take a full-on, deep dive. We are going to get right into the finer details regarding what we should be eating and how we should be working out if we are going to take care of our guts.

It is going to be a fun one. So don't touch that dial.

Chapter 7:
Eating for Your Gut—the Role of Diet and Exercise

If we are being honest, I think we can all say that the whole concept of "diet" is getting a little played out.

Fad diets have been around forever, certainly, but do they not seem to be getting more prevalent all the time? Have we not lived through maybe the most prolific period in the history of these things?

Just think of how many we have seen in the last 20 years. And then think of all the conflicting evidence, all the anecdotal success stories, and the way they seem to spread like mind viruses. It is a bizarre phenomenon; I will say that.

But I think what lies at the center of them is that we are all aware that what we eat matters. Especially in North America, we know that our diets are not sustainable. We know that we should take better care of ourselves, not eat enormous bags of chips as a meal, and not drink eight liters of cola a day. And even in a less extreme place, we know that we should be eating more fruits and vegetables, more whole grains—the whole gamut.

So, there is a positive to all this searching for the perfect diet. It is a conscious effort on our part to change our ways in order to be healthier.

The negative to them, however, is obvious: Most of them are based on flimsy premises, usually with a grain of truth that gets extrapolated into another dimension. And they reveal another fundamental truth about our species, which is that we tend to look for the easy way out.

Which is kind of the fad diet in a nutshell, no? An easy way to allegedly get healthy is based on faulty premises.

What I am saying here is that I do not want to recommend some fad diet. I want to be honest about what it takes to eat healthily, and I want to use the best science available to make this recommendation. I want to admit that, yes, it is going to take some doing to pull off a healthy diet. But, according to research, it is not only possible but imperative that you do so.

What I want to do here is really get into the *why* of things. Let's talk about some of the research around protein, fats, and carbs, as well as probiotics and prebiotics, and let's really try to dig deep and understand how these things are affecting our gut health.

Hopefully, by the time this chapter is over, I will have convinced you that dieting for gut health is not just a fad. This is the real deal.

And when that is done? Well, we are going to get into some exercise. We are going to talk about why it is important for our guts, and we are going to talk about some exercises we should be doing to make gut health happen.

So, let's get started.

Protein

The effect that dietary protein has on gut microbiota was first observed and recorded as far back as 1977. Since then, a whole boatload of studies have come out, looking at everything from animal-based proteins, including eggs, to whey protein and vegetarian protein (Singh *et al.*, 2017).

All of them have confirmed that there is a positive correlation between protein consumption and the diversity of your gut microbiome. Even the humble pea protein was found to increase the presence of a microbe that works as an anti-inflammatory.

In other words, protein is an essential ingredient for maintaining gut health. Which, for some of you, might indicate further evidence that the keto diet is a good option for your health.

But you would be wrong, alas. In fact, while high-protein and low-carb diets are associated with weight loss, they do horrific things to your gut microbiome. And additionally, high amounts of proteins found in red meat have been found to increase a type of bacteria that is positively associated with cardiovascular disease.

So, it is not just a high-protein diet that is important. Where you get that protein from matters, as does whether or not it is part of a balanced diet.

This has been confirmed in mouse studies, where intakes of plant-based protein showed a lesser risk of cancer and diabetes and an overall trend toward early death. So, the humble pea protein might be lifting above its weight class even more than we thought.

Fats

By now, we all know that diets high in saturated and trans fats are wicked bad for us. They cause all manner of bad things, from cancer to heart attacks to everything in between. We also know that the Western diet, so-called, is high in both of these things.

But fat is nonetheless good for us. We need them for all kinds of things. We especially need mono- and polyunsaturated fats, both of which lead to a *decreased* risk of chronic disease (Singh *et al.*, 2017).

In addition to all this, fats of all stripes affect our gut microflora. Considering the binary we have of saturated and trans fats being bad for us and mono- and polyunsaturated fats being good for us, what are the odds that this also holds true when it comes to the gut microbiome?

As it turns out, this is exactly the truth. And not only has this held true in animal studies—in this case, studies done on rats—but in human-based trials, too. For example, when rats were given lard, there was an increase in unhealthy bacteria, and when they were given fish oil, there was an increase in healthy bacteria.

So, while the plant-based protein, in general, promoted an increase in gut health greater than animal-based protein, fish oil-derived fats were better for our guts than lard, which comes from pigs. There is a pattern here related to animal products that I am not going to explicitly weigh in on, but it does appear, so far, as though pescatarian diets might be best for our guts...?

Carbs

Here, we are going to get into two different types of carbs: The digestible kind (starch, sugars) and the indigestible kind (fiber).

So, with regard to...

Digestible Carbs

If we are perceptive, we will have noticed a pattern and likely be able to predict what is coming under this subheading.

Sugars that come from fruits promote healthy bacteria; sugars that come from candies and the like promote unhealthy bacteria (Singh *et al.*, 2017). Controversially, though, lactose, while most commonly understood as an irritant to the digestive system, appears to promote healthy bacteria. Why is this? Well, the study admits that it does not understand these findings. So, we will have to flag that for now.

But the findings around artificial sweeteners are maybe even more controversial than this. The findings state that artificial sweeteners might, in fact, be *more* unhealthy than natural sugars, which is not how they were understood even a few years ago. In fact, they were talked about as a no-calorie solution to a supposed sugar problem.

Alas, the effect they have on our gut bacterial cultures is almost entirely negative and leads to a greater risk of glucose intolerance. So, they should be avoided when possible.

Alright. So much for digestible carbs. On to...

Non-Digestible Carbs (Fiber)

By now, we should know that fiber refers to non-digestible matter, which helps move things along in your digestive system. Not eating fiber means, frankly, you are going to have trouble pooping. Eating plenty means allowing things to exit regularly.

But in addition to this, fiber also ferments in the digestive system. In doing so, it "modifies the intestinal environment" in such a way to technically qualify as a prebiotic. So here we can talk about soybeans, raw oats, and unrefined wheat and barley (Singh *et al.*, 2017).

So, what does this mean for gut health? Well, studies have shown that diets that lack these substances actually reduce bacterial abundance. And what is more, another study looked at 49 obese subjects, provided them with a high intake of fiber, and then studied their gut culture diversity.

It will come as no surprise that the fiber-rich diet led to a healthier gut by increasing the amount of good bacteria in it. These kinds of bacteria, too, would lead to greater immune function and a healthier metabolism. Which means that at least some of the health problems associated with obesity can be countered by a fiber-rich diet.

And as if that is not cool enough, it also appears to lead to reductions in body weight. Which sheds light on at least one dietary change we need to make, provided weight loss is one of our goals.

Probiotics

These have been covered at length elsewhere, so I will only briefly glance over them this time. But these types of fermented foods promote healthy gut bacteria, full stop, and are an integral part of this process of keeping healthy guts.

We know what they include, but for a refresher: yogurt, kimchi, sauerkraut, et cetera.

The benefits of consuming these products are legion. They include alleviating GI intolerance symptoms, accelerating what is called "intestinal transit time" (which I am pretty sure you can translate yourself), and decreasing abdominal distention in people with chronic liver problems (Singh *et al.*, 2017).

And as if that were not enough, it also helps with traveler's diarrhea. So that's nice.

But as I said, we have already covered probiotics, so I will not spend more time going over what we already know. Suffice it to say that consuming them is a key ingredient in our overall health and is wholeheartedly recommended.

***

Alright, so if we are being super honest, the fact that diet and gut health are connected does not exactly require a leap of imagination. It is pretty clear that what we eat affects the part of our body that digests what we eat. So, in that sense, I assume you really did not need me to get too deep with that information.

But the thing I wanted to stress here is that while there are certain required elements for our gut health, like, say, protein, not all of these things are created equal. Protein from vegetable products is better for our gut health than what we get from animals. And the fats we get from fish are better than those we get from pigs.

And so on, for virtually every aspect of our diet. Which is interesting to me because, while we often talk about diabetes and obesity, unhealthy food choices affect every area of our health. Unhealthy sugar sources also play havoc with our guts, which in turn affects our immune systems, which leads to us getting sick.

Basically, our body is a kind of machine that requires everything to be in sync. We need good fuel sources in order for everything in our body to work well. Our guts are a significant part of this, but the solution to gut health is the same as it is for everything: Eat plenty of fiber, go easy on the red meat, get your sugars from whole grains and fruit, and so on.

Which is why it should come as no surprise that the next half of this chapter is going to focus on exercise. Because, yes, diet and exercise are the two main ingredients when it comes to being healthy.

And whether we are talking about obesity, heart health, mental health, or gut health, this is always going to be a constant.

But let's get into the weeds here with exercise and gut health and see what we can't find out!

Exercise

Okay, so while a few of the topics in this book have begun with me admitting that the research on this or that thing is scarce, this is not so with exercise and gut health. The research is as clear as it can be, with even just six weeks of exercising having been shown to positively impact overall gut health (Pratt, 2018).

And by the way, this benefit occurs independent of diet or any other factors. How they did this was that they took people who were lean and people who were obese, measured their microbiomes, and then put them on an exercise regimen. This regimen involved 30–40 minutes of cardio three times a week for six weeks. Once this was done, they measured their gut microbiomes again.

What they found will not be surprising to us by now. There was a definite change in which bacteria were present in their guts: Some of them increased, and some of them decreased. The ones that increased were positively associated with lower risks of heart disease, type 2 diabetes, and obesity.

And then, just to make sure, the researchers had the participants return to their pre-exercise, sedentary lifestyles. Once this was done, their bacterial cultures returned to the levels they had been at prior to introducing regular exercise.

So, what does this mean?

First off, you can't just exercise for six weeks and then accrue the benefits. Exercise has to be maintained, or else the unhealthy bacteria will again be in the ascendant.

But additionally, the benefits of long-term exercise are not known. Does exercising for longer periods produce greater results? Or is there a plateau? If there is a plateau, at which point does it occur?

This is an interesting field to be in right now because it is only recently that there has been any interest in it at all. But all of a sudden, it has proven itself to be fertile ground for research, which suggests that more information will be coming in with greater frequency.

Already, gut health has been shown to affect diseases like obesity and depression, among others. However, the research also shows that gut health and IBS are linked, as well as inflammatory bowel disease. So, what does this mean for the role of exercise in treating these ailments?

Put simply, exercise is only one component of treatment, but it is a significant one. The effect that it has on symptoms is that it assists in alleviating them, particularly when a consistent exercise regimen is adopted and not abandoned. So, a consistent exercise regimen, in addition to whichever other therapeutic interventions are necessary, is going to help heal the body if any of these ailments are present.

A lot of Latinate words for a simple idea: Exercise is good for you, so you should do it.

But which exercises should you be doing? Well, am I ever glad you asked?

Sample Exercises for Gut Health

The first thing we should have noticed in the above section is that the study was performed on patients using cardiovascular exercise. So, which cardio exercises should we be doing to maximize gut health?

"Cardio" is basically any exercise that works out our hearts and lungs. This means running, skipping, jumping jacks—anything that gets our hearts moving and our lungs breathing.

Since the study focused on 30-minute exercise periods, this is going to be my recommendation as well. This means that three days a week, we should be doing some kind of exercise that brings us close to being out of breath.

And which kinds are those?

Brisk Walking

This sounds like a stupid one, but especially for beginners, this is a fantastic way to get the blood moving. Most of us have to walk throughout the day, although that is probably less now that so many of us work from home. But even if it is going to the grocery store or going uptown to see a movie, whatever it is you need to walk to, try doing it at a brisk pace and see where that gets you.

Once you get comfortable with this, set aside 30 minutes a day, three days a week, with a specific destination in mind. You will be feeling the effects of this exercise in no time.

But if you are more advanced?

Running

This is a great exercise, no matter who you are. There are so many benefits to running, including the oft-cited "runner's high" that comes at the end. It is, really, an excellent way to help get yourself in shape, provided you know how to do it safely.

Because, yes, there is the possibility that you might hurt yourself. But really, we all know how to run instinctively. Just make sure you listen to your body, have a good pair of shoes, and try not to push yourself to the breaking point when you do not have to.

The other cool thing about running, though, is that you can do it outdoors or on a treadmill. I am not much of an outdoor cat, so I like to use the treadmill. But to each their own! If running outside is your bag, then go for it.

Additionally, if you are just starting out, then do not feel bad if you cannot do 30 minutes at a time. Remember, that is the goal, not the starting point. If you have to work your way up to 30 minutes of continuous exercise, then by all means, do so.

But maybe you are finding that running isn't your thing. Maybe you prefer something with a little more speed. In that case...

Cycling

This is another one you can do indoors or outdoors. And no, I do not mean that you can ride your bicycle around inside. That would be a bad idea.

What I mean is that the stationary bike is a great little invention. And why is this? Well, take me, for instance. I live in a city. Biking in a big city takes a type of courage I do not have. People do it all the time and bless 'em. But me? I did it once, and that was enough.

For me, then, the stationary bike is a godsend. I like how you can adjust it to different levels of difficulty, how you can get it to pretend you are going uphill, then downhill, and how it adjusts the resistance on its own... Anyway, I sound like I am gushing, I know. But I like this instrument.

Still, whether you do it indoors or outdoors, cycling is excellent for your cardio. And thereby excellent for your gut health.

***

So much for cardio. But by now, we might be asking, Is weight training important for gut health too?

While the study we referred to discussed the impact of cardio on the gut, weight training is an important part of exercise, no matter what. In fact, one of the benefits of weight training is that it helps your body handle the stress of regular exercise. Which means you can work out more often.

So, is weight training recommended? Absolutely. And here are some exercises I personally suggest you try adopting:

Free Weights

Any exercise where you are using a weight that is not tethered to a machine is a free weight. This means dumbbells, barbells, even cowbells (just kidding—no cowbell).

With these types of weights, you can do a whole bunch of exercises, all of which focus on different muscle groups. You can do bicep curls, lunges, deadlifts, bench presses, etc. You can even do more complicated ones where multiple movements are required to complete the repetition.

No matter what, "repetition" is the key part of free-weight exercises. A repetition is defined simply as completing the exercise once. So, for a bicep curl, it means raising and lowering your arm one time. A "set" is the number of repetitions required to complete that set; so, for example, you might do one set of 10 repetitions. From there, you probably do three sets, which means, in total, 30 repetitions.

Different exercises require different numbers of sets and reps, depending on what your goals are.

Anyway, one of the benefits of free-weight exercises is that they require you to stabilize your body in such a way that more parts of it get worked out than whatever you are focusing on. So even doing bicep curls winds up working out your abdominals, for example, simply because you are trying to keep upright and not slouch.

But because of this, there are also dangers to using them. It is much easier to get hurt, even from such a simple thing as dropping the weights.

For that reason, some people are more attracted to...

Machines

Firstly, machines are great. If you do not believe me, look at someone like Arnold. The dude loves his machines. And not just because he is the Terminator, either. Every workout video I see of that guy tends to be using one or the other machine.

Basically, how these work is that each machine has something you push or pull that is attached to a number of weights. You set the weight you are comfortable with and then do however many reps and sets you have decided you want to.

The benefit of machines is that they technically do the stabilizing for you. You are way less likely to get hurt using them (although getting hurt is still possible) since there is little worry about, say, dropping the weight on yourself.

And, since they do most of the stabilizing for you, they also help you isolate whichever muscle group you want to work on. In other words, if you are doing a pull-down exercise, you are really targeting your back and arms. Which is a bit of a good and bad thing, depending on what your goals are.

Nonetheless, machines are a great way to work out. They are generally safer than free weights; there are plenty of options at the gym; and in many cases, they might be the best thing available for doing a particular type of exercise.

So, absolutely make machine workouts a part of your routine.

***

Alright. Time for a summary.

What you eat and how you move your body matter. Both of those things do. And not just in the sense that they help keep you lean and in shape or because they help prevent diabetes and cardiac problems. They have a significant influence on our guts. And since our guts are connected to everything from brain health to immune function, these two activities matter way more than they might even appear at first glance—and that is saying something.

Crucially, the types of nutrients we take in and where we take them matter a whole lot. We know now that different types of fats have different effects on our guts. That different types of sugars do too. So, we need to be conscious of where we get these things from when we are, say, at the grocery store.

Fortunately, we all have a pretty good idea of what is healthy and what is not. The interesting thing is that unhealthy food has a negative effect on virtually every part of our bodies. Sugary candies are bad for our teeth, our glucose and insulin levels, and, as it turns out, for our digestive systems. Bad food really does swing a lot of weight around.

But eating healthy is not the only solution to this problem. We know now that exercise, especially cardio, has a positive effect on our gut health, resulting in higher quantities of healthy bacteria. But we also know that regular exercise has to be maintained and that we can't do it for a while, stop, and continue to reap the benefits.

Exercise has to be done at least three days a week, for 30 minutes or more at a time. If we can do that, the benefits will follow.

So much for diet and exercise. What else is there?

Myths.

No, not the Greco-Roman kind. Although those are awesome. No, I mean common myths about gut health. Persistent errors, both factual and rational, have continuously dogged our understanding.

It's time to clear those up.

Chapter 8:
Myths and Truths—FAQs

Yes, that is right: It is time to tackle the common myths around gut health.

This is the main event, ladies and gentlemen. Me versus the untruths. One-on-one. *Mano a mano.* All those little non-facts we have running around in our noodles were finally brought to light and wrecked in the ultimate heavyweight battle for factual supremacy.

Alright, so I've been watching a lot of wrestling lately. Still, every one of us has these nuggets of untruth roiling away in our subconsciousness, and they are mostly innocuous. But today, we are going to tackle them one at a time because I think knowing the truth is better than the alternative.

So here we go: The common myths around gut health, finally debunked.

Myth #1: You Should Poop Every Day

This sounds kind of dumb, right? It is almost like saying, "It is a common myth that you should breathe every day." Everybody, as the storybook says, poops. Even Jill Biden—so, of course, we should do it every day.

And yeah, technically. But only for some people! In fact, depending on hydration, stress, and a whole host of other things, you might only use Number 2 three times a week (Carver-Carter, 2022).

Which sounds like it is not a lot. But really, the only thing that should worry you is if there is a drastic change in your schedule. Or if your current schedule causes you some level of discomfort. In that case, you can always talk to a doctor, who remains the resident expert in these matters.

Let me put it to you this way. You know how there is always that kid at school who seems to catch onto everything super quickly? And he gets everything he wants because he is kind of a natural? Well, for lots of people, this person is a sign of their own inadequacies. They look at him and say, "How come I'm not getting into medical school at 19?" They see it as a sign of failure—in other words that they are not on the same schedule as this guy.

Well, guess what? Everyone has their own schedule. Every person does this or that thing at different times, and that is okay. Some people take a year off after high school to work and figure themselves out. Some people do not.

Some people poop every day. Others do not. The Judeo-Christian tradition has a commandment that quite clearly says not to look into your neighbor's yard and desire what he has—his wife, his ox, whatever. Well, this goes for pooping as well. Do not covet another man's pooping schedule. It makes no sense.

Myth #2: Stress Causes Stomach Ulcers

You read that correctly. It is a myth that stress causes stomach ulcers.

Now, the story of how this was discovered is interesting. An Australian scientist named Barry Marshall theorized that *H pylori*, a bacterium, was not only pathogenic but responsible for stomach ulcers (Marshall, Adams, 2008). He encountered a brick wall of skepticism, however, which for two years seemed impossible to bypass.

So, what could he possibly do to overcome this? There were no animal studies proving his theory. The theory itself was not catching on the way he had hoped. What was left?

The biological sciences are filled with instances of scientists ingesting pathogens or otherwise turning themselves into research participants on whom to test their theories, which is odd but true. The man who discovered the plague vaccines, for example, first injected himself with them to prove that they worked.

Another notable self-experimenter was a man named John Hunter, who injected himself with gonorrhea and syphilis (Moore, 2009). This man was considered to be the greatest surgeon in London—or, at least, the most highly paid. He had a theory that gonorrhea and syphilis were, in fact, the same illness and insisted on proving it via self-experimentation.

The problem is that Hunter injected himself with gonorrhea but *accidentally* also injected himself with syphilis, since the needle had been infected with the latter disease and had not been cleaned but instead reused by Hunter. So, he had both diseases at once, and this led him to say that his theories had been right, although only because he unknowingly made a mistake.

Interesting fact about John Hunter: He was a teacher, specifically in anatomy. Every day, his students would arrive at the lab to find a cadaver on a gurney, which he would lead them in dissecting. The day of his death, however, his instructions were that his own body be placed on the gurney so that his students could dissect him. It was, he thought, his final gift to them.

But that is neither here nor there. Back to Barry Marshall.

By now, you can see where this is going, no? What Barry Marshall did was collect a bacterial culture from a patient with dyspepsia (Marshall, Adams, 2008). He then ingested the bacterial culture himself, followed by regular testing.

So again, the theory was that anyone was susceptible to *H pylori*, and that, if infected, this would lead to gastritis and maybe, years later, ulcers, which ran against conventional wisdom.

What he found after infecting himself was that he was bloated, and every morning he vomited clear liquid, without bile. He had gastritis, which proved his theory. He began taking antibiotics at his wife's insistence, although he thinks the infection may have cleared up on its own. And in any case, the infection was done away with, and he was right.

For his efforts, he was awarded the Nobel Prize. Which seems like a sensible reward for doing such a crazy thing. In any case, we have further evidence that unhealthy bacteria in our guts are bad for us and should be kept in check. Diet and exercise and all that, right?

Which leads us to our next myth...

Myth #3: All Bacteria Are Bad for Us

The reason why we think of sickness when we think of bacteria is not for nothing. Bacterial infections can be a real nightmare.

Consider the following: pneumonia; meningitis, strep throat, food poisoning. All of them have two things in common. They all *suck*, and they are all types of illnesses caused by bacterial infections.

For myself, I have had both strep throat and food poisoning. The last time I had strep would have been the sickest I had ever been until the time I got food poisoning.

For the strep, it was the usual story. I was out with some friends—in fact, I was doing karaoke. And then, all of a sudden, there was this awful pain in my throat and a feeling like I was dehydrated. Obviously, I was drinking at the time, so I put it down to that.

But when I got up the next morning, I felt wretched. I decided to look in the mirror to see the back of my throat, almost on a whim. And there it was: The telltale duo of white lines along the back.

It took a while before I felt better. I took antibiotics, and I rested up a whole bit. But the feeling was terrible. No amount of cold water could soothe my throat. No amount of lozenges, nothing. Just pain until it was over.

And about food poisoning? Well, the less said about it, the better. Suffice it to say, it involved late-night chicken wings that, as it turns out, were undercooked. I wound up with salmonella that lasted a week and a half.

Awful, awful experiences—and both of them are due to bacterial infections.

But this is obviously only part of the picture. Think of all we have talked about already—probiotics, for example. We have all these bacteria in our intestines, our colon, which we need in order to survive.

"Bacteria" refers to an entire domain of life. This means it is distinguished from eukaryotes, which include all animals, plants, and fungi, and archaea, which is another type of unicellular life form. In other words, if under eukaryotes, we have all animals and plants, just for starters, think of how diverse the eukaryotes are. Maybe bacteria are not as diverse as that; maybe they are—but there is a significant level of diversity within that domain. And just like some mushrooms are healthy, some get you high, and some kill you, not all bacteria make you sick.

Anyway, you get the idea. Do not be afraid of bacteria; only some kinds.

Myth #4: Gluten Is Bad for Your Gut

I am going to get into fad diets more specifically in a second. But was there any diet more faddish in our lifetime than the push for gluten-free everything?

Before I get into this, I want to be clear: Gluten allergies are, of course, a real thing. Celiac disease is a terrible ailment, and sufferers really do have quite the time of it. So, when I say that the push for gluten-free everything was a fad, by no means am I saying that celiac disease is a part of that. In fact, having gluten-free options available for people with celiac disease is a good thing.

But.

Most of us not only do not have a gluten intolerance but also need gluten in order to get a whole bunch of essential nutrients. It is just not the case that gluten is unhealthy for us overall. It is a problem for people with an allergy to it or even to wheat products.

So, let's get into this a bit, then. First off, we should define what gluten is, so we know we are on the same page. And then, we will run over why it is not something we should be worried about.

When we think of "gluten," we might be thinking of a single substance. But it actually refers to a whole bunch of things, all of them proteins, which are found in wheat, barley, rye, and triticale (Kubala, 2019).

The thing about gluten proteins is that they are very elastic, which is why grains that contain gluten are best for bread-making or for making other baked goods. This is so true that, for many baked goods, a powdery substance known as wheat gluten is often added to give the baked goods extra rise and strength.

And yet, some people do develop an intolerance to gluten. This comes in three varieties, which we will go into one at a time.

The first is perhaps the most widely known and is called "celiac disease." This affects somewhere around 1% of the population, although in Finland, Mexico, and North Africa, that number is somewhere around 2–5%.

The disease itself is an inflammatory bowel disease, specifically of the small intestine. What happens is that the gluten damages the cells lining the intestinal wall, which can cause malabsorption of nutrients as well as diarrhea. Additionally, people with celiac disease may have anemia, neurological disorders, and dermatitis. And then, some people might be totally asymptomatic.

Celiac disease is diagnosed via intestinal biopsy or blood testing.

Next up is a good ol' fashioned wheat allergy. This tends to affect children, but some adults also have it. The symptoms of a wheat allergy are the basic allergy symptoms, from nausea and discomfort all the way to anaphylaxis.

This is diagnosed via skin-prick testing.

There is also non-celiac gluten sensitivity, which is when someone without celiac or a wheat allergy experiences discomfort after ingesting gluten. It can only be diagnosed when those other two are ruled out, and even then, as a diagnosis, it appears to be controversial, particularly since it relies so much on self-reporting. We will get back to this in a second.

Okay, so much for the varieties of gluten sensitivity. The question then is: Should the population outside of these demographics cut back on, or refrain from entirely, gluten-containing products? And if not, then why do some people report feeling better when they go on a gluten-free diet?

Let's start with the second question first. There are a few reasons why some people might report feeling better when they go gluten-free but think of the kinds of products that would contain gluten to begin with for a clue.

Pizza. Beer. Bagels. Pastries.

If we are the kind of person who eats a boatload of these things, we probably feel sick without even noticing it. Cutting back on this kind of food is, of course, going to make you feel better. Who would not feel better after having cut back on pizza and beer?

Which is where we come back to non-celiac gluten sensitivity. A lot of the self-reporting comes from people saying they feel tired, that their joints ache, and that their mood stinks. But there is a big question at the center of these symptoms: Why is it that they are identical to symptoms of a diet high in refined carbs and sugars?

Is it possible that the reason it remains medically unrecognized is that some people are just eating too much pizza and blaming their sluggish, angry states on the gluten?

Well, look, I am not one to weigh in on this, I know. And while I think I have shown my hand, I will admit that there are people out there who know way more than I do. So, take what I say with a grain of salt.

Furthermore, there is no reason to think that a gluten-free diet is *unhealthy* for someone without an intolerance to the stuff. It is just a question of whether or not it is necessary. And since there is no harm in cutting it out, then that would be up to you.

Myth #5: [Insert Fad Diet Here] Works!

This is a bit of a broad one, but I promise it is connected.

I have previously mentioned my distaste for fad diets. They tend not to rely on science, for starters, and make all kinds of promises they cannot keep. They are much more akin to snake oil than an actual remedy for good health.

And yet, 45 million Americans will "go on a diet" every year (Kingsley, 2023). It is a trend—albeit starting with much smaller numbers—that began as far back as the 19th century when dieting culture first entered the United States. Since then, all it has ever taken to get one of these things going is for a single element to enter the culture: Anything from a new scientific finding around this or that nutrient to a lone wolf doctor claiming he has found the key to our long-lasting good health.

The first guy to set off a dieting fad in the U.S. that resembles the kinds of dieting fads we have now was a Presbyterian minister named Sylvester Graham. This fellow was on a tear about how processed flours would damage your health and produced his own strain from wheat germ instead of endosperm, which was the usual way of making this stuff.

Since then, there have been a whole host of weird things people have come up with as a means of unlocking their health. One of these included "floor-rolling," where people would literally just roll around on the floor. Others would eat nothing but skim milk and bananas. Still, more would give themselves yogurt enemas.

In the mid-1800's, there was a guy named Banting who promoted a low-carb diet. This is interesting to me because it shows how long we have been scared of carbs. There was even a period where people would have these weird roller-things rubbed all over their bodies, supposedly to lose weight through the power of electricity.

For my money, the grossest of all these would be the "cabbage soup diet," where people would eat as much of the stuff as they could get their hands on. Who the heck would ever want to eat that much cabbage soup? At least skim milk and bananas would be tasty the first few times. But *cabbage soup?*

Then, of course, there was Mr. Atkins, who promoted a low-carb, high-fat diet. This would be resurrected all those years later as the "keto diet," which was literally the exact same thing. Atkins even talked about sending the body into ketosis. But of course, these things come in waves and cycles, and people have short memories.

Anyway, I could go on with all the different weird things people have done to hack their way into good health. But the point here is this: None of these methods worked. Not that there was not some grain of truth to them. Of course, there were! Nothing in the world can be convincing without being at least kind of true.

The problem was that whatever was true about them was not their conclusion. Is cabbage soup good for you? Sure, probably. Maybe it even has some weight-loss properties. We have certainly seen in this book that promoting certain types of gut bacteria is associated with higher metabolism and so forth. But does that mean that stuffing ourselves with it is going to magically make us fit, happy, and sane?

No, these diet fads are myths. If we are going to adopt behaviors that promote good health, they are not going to be via some quick and easy hack. They are going to involve diet and exercise, and a balanced diet, to boot.

However we proceed, whatever we proceed with, we should make sure that it is backed by solid science. And we should be wary of claims about there being a secret ingredient that will make us lean with no extra work put in. This is a telltale sign that the proposal is not based on fact.

Know the signs. Remember, if it sounds too good to be true it probably is.

Myth #6: Chewing Gum Will Sit In Your Stomach for 7 Years

Alright, this is a fun one to laugh at, *but who among us did not, at some point think this was true?*

I mean, sure, it makes no sense. Of course, gum passes through the body just the same way everything else does. But did we not, all of us, at some point, imagine our stomachs dotted with all the chewing gum we swallowed over the years? I even remember it being in a cartoon—maybe *Hey Arnold* or something. It was a close-up X-ray shot of someone's stomach, where the lining was dotted with swallowed gum. Maybe *Ren and Stimpy*?

Anyway, that is not important. The important thing is that this is a myth. *It is not true!* Sure, chewing gum may not technically be super good for you. But swallowing it is not going to lead to seven years of indigestible, rubbery material stuck inside our bodies.

But is there even a grain of truth to this?

Well, as it turns out, while many of the ingredients, including the sweeteners, preservatives, and the like, are perfectly digestible, the actual gum base is not (Santos-Longhurst, 2018). Traditionally, this was made out of a kind of sap. But people do like chewing gum, and so the demand increased, which meant the race was on to find a base that was not as challenging to get a hold of.

This is why, nowadays, chewing gum is made up of synthetic polymers. But like lots of other indigestible matter, including fiber, gum will not sit in your stomach for more than a few days.

Notice, too, that I compared chewing gum to fiber. While it is certainly not healthy in the same way that fiber is, it is nonetheless true that our bodies process material that is technically indigestible all the time.

The most obvious example of this is corn. Without getting too graphic, we have all become aware at one time or another that corn shells are not digested and are excreted more or less intact. Chewing gum, as long as it is not an enormous piece that is going to cause you trouble, will come out pretty well in the exact same way.

In fact, gum will go through all the stages you would expect anything else you eat to go through. You put it in your mouth; you chew it until the flavor runs out; ideally, you spit it out, but for this example, you swallow it; it goes down your esophagus and into your stomach; from there, it enters your small intestine; your small intestine absorbs whatever nutrients are available from the gum, including sugars; what is indigestible in the gum moves into your colon; then passes through your rectum during a bowel movement, only to flush away into oblivion.

The whole process will, for sure, take less than seven days. Which is considerably less than the seven years it is supposed to sit in your stomach for—wherever that number came from, God only knows.

Now, all of this makes swallowing gum seem harmless. But is it?

Well, not exactly. Swallowing large amounts of gum can cause certain problems. This includes whether it is swallowed all at once or over a long period of time. If this happens, it can form what is known as a "bezoar."

And what is a bezoar? Well, am I ever glad you asked.

A bezoar is more than just a cool name. It refers to a lump of undigested material that accumulates in the gastrointestinal system, usually in the stomach (WebMD Editorial Contributors, 2023). This can cause a blockage in the small intestine, which may or may not result in problems down the road. Most of these are asymptomatic; some of them are not.

There are a few types of these wild things, and we are going to go over a few of them here:

The first is called a lactobezoar. This is predominantly found in milk-fed infants and is made up of milk protein and mucus.

There are foreign body bezoars too. These are from things like parasitic worms, plastic, and polystyrene foam cups, which means, yes, that some people eat those cups.

Phytobezoars are made up of indigestible food fibers. This is the most common type and is mostly created by fruits and vegetables, like pumpkins, sunflower seeds, and raisins.

Trichobezoars are, in essence, hairballs. They can develop into what is known as "Rapunzel syndrome," where the hairball winds up, forming a tail that extends into the small intestine. This typically affects adolescent girls, but people with developmental disabilities and psychiatric disorders are also at risk.

Specifically, any overeating of indigestible matter puts you at risk of getting one of these things. But there are some people who are more likely to do this than others.

Certain behavioral disorders may compel someone to do this. "Pica" is a well-known example where people compulsively eat non-nutritive matter, like rocks. But some people have something as simple as an altered gastrointestinal anatomy, which makes them more likely to get a bezoar. It is the same as people who have to breathe through ventilation, have problems chewing food either because they use dentures, do not have teeth, or have reduced stomach size, say, from surgery.

Again, most of these do not develop symptoms at all. But in cases where they do, there are some common ones.

A lack of appetite is common and understandable. It is hard to feel hungry when your stomach is blocked. But even if you do have an appetite, you might find that you are full after only eating a small amount. This can lead to weight loss, but not in a good way.

Vomiting and abdominal pain are also symptoms. Same as bloating and anemia.

They can also put a strain on your digestive system, causing internal bleeding. If this happens, you may find blood in your stool. There is also a risk that they may cause one portion of your intestines to wrap around another, cutting off the blood supply. If this happens, a portion of your intestines may die. This is called intussusception.

There is also a not-super-high risk that they may cause intestinal perforation. If that happens, digestive fluids may leak into the abdomen, causing bloating and severe pain that goes all the way up to your shoulder. This is considered a medical emergency and should be dealt with immediately by a doctor.

Luckily, they are treatable. There are medications we can take to dissolve them, but if they are too big for that, then surgery may be recommended.

An interesting fact about bezoars: For the longest time, bezoars found in animals were highly valued and believed to have magic properties (Fick n.d.). In fact, the word bezoar comes from a Persian word that means "antidote." They were found in the stomachs of animals that had just been sacrificed (this is from a long time ago, obviously), and in smooth, round shapes that were often quite beautiful to look at.

Among the things they were assumed to cure were leprosy, measles, cholera, and depression. They were also worn as charms and were said to cure poison.

Arabian doctors were the ones who brought them into Europe in the 12th century, where they were offered as cures for arsenic—the poison most used to kill aristocrats and royalty. They became super big business, so much so that by the 16th century, they were worth 10 times their weight in gold, and Queen Elizabeth I wore one in a silver ring.

Knockoffs became popular too. Jesuit priests made a bunch of bezoar-like things called Goa stones, which were said to cure poison and the plague. And it was not until much later, through a gruesome series of events, that bezoars were discovered to not have healing properties at all.

What happened was that, in 1575, a French nobleman caught his cook stealing his silver. The cook was given the death penalty, and a hanging was set. However, the Frenchman, a fellow named Paré, was interested in testing the healing properties of bezoars, and so he struck a deal with him.

The deal was that if the cook agreed to take a lethal dose of poison, Paré would use a bezoar on him to see if it worked as a cure. If it worked, the cook was free to go. If it did not, the cook would die.

Now, I have no idea if death by poison is worse than death by hanging. But the cook, living in a time during which bezoars were widely assumed to be an antidote to poison, surely must have seen this as the easiest deal he had ever made.

He agreed to take the poison, of course. However, bezoars do not have healing properties, nor are they an antidote to anything. Paré attempted to administer the bezoar, and the cook died. Thus, it was discovered that bezoars are not medicinal, nor are they curative.

All of which is to say: Okay, sure, chewing gum does not sit in your stomach for seven years. But if you swallow too much of it too often, you could get one of these nasty bezoar things. And since they are not much good for anything outside of blocking your intestines and making you vomit, it is a good idea to stay away from the habit of swallowing gum anyway.

Myth #7: Eating Before Bed Is Bad for You

This one is getting a "partly true" rating from me. Conventional wisdom, however, says that eating before bed is responsible for not only weight gain but also nightmares. That last one I had heard all the time from my mom when I was a kid. But as far as weight gain?

Well, as we will see, eating before bed might affect our guts in an undesirable way. Just maybe not in the way we thought.

So, the reason why some people say eating before bed causes you to gain weight is because your metabolism, supposedly, slows down while you sleep. Using some deductive reasoning here, having food in our stomachs while our metabolism is taking a breather would mean not breaking the food down as efficiently. Which, it follows, would mean weight gain.

Conversely, there are some people out there claiming that the *opposite* is true. They say that eating before bed will not only help you sleep better but will actually lead to weight *loss*.

Is either one of these true? Or is the answer somewhere in between?

First off, your metabolism actually does not slow down while you sleep—at least not significantly (Jones, 2023). As it turns out, you need energy while you sleep too. So, while there is a slight drop-off in your baseline metabolic rate, it is not enough to make eating before bed a cause of weight gain in itself.

And yet, bedtime eating is a trait often found in people who are overweight. *But why?*

The answer is a lot simpler than you might think. Essentially, people who eat before bed often have bad eating habits to begin with. They tend to be—although not universally—people who have problems with diet and, we can speculate, might be eating before bed to satisfy food cravings rather than genuine hunger.

Oftentimes, as it turns out, we are not talking about people who have a snack before bed but who eat an entire meal, which means, as an extra meal, taking in that many more calories.

Which might be normal for, say, a bodybuilder. Or a powerlifter. But unless there is an athletic reason that requires us to eat an extra meal, having that extra meal is only going to mean going well over our daily caloric recommendations.

Another thing is that people who skip meals tend to be hungriest just before bed. This means they eat a bunch before they sleep, wake up not feeling hungry, skip breakfast, and so on.

This cycle can lead to weight gain. But luckily, it can be fixed by eating balanced meals throughout the day, which is nice and easy.

But since we are here to talk about gut health and not eating disorders, let's pivot for a second. Because one type of person who will want to avoid eating before bed, maybe more than anyone else, is someone who suffers from acid reflux.

Gastroesophageal reflux disease (GERD) affects somewhere between 18 and 28% of Americans. Basically, what happens is that your stomach acid "splashes back" into your throat, which causes a whole bunch of undesirable symptoms.

What might those symptoms be? Well, heartburn may be the one most commonly associated with it. But it also presents as a lump in the throat, difficulty swallowing, dental erosions, and laryngitis.

As far as diseases of the gut go, it is not a fun one. (As if there are any!) But the problem with eating before bed is that since you are lying down, it is easier to regurgitate, which means your acid reflux is going to get a whole lot worse.

For people with GERD, then, eating before bed is not recommended. But while I have you here, there are some studies that seem to show that having a light snack before bed really does help you sleep better. And also might stabilize your morning blood sugar.

Both of these things are going to be good for your gut health. So do not write off eating before bed entirely!

Myth #8: "Leaky Gut" Results in Food Particles Entering Your Bloodstream

There are a couple of things to cover here. So first, I am going to start with a leaky gut and then get into this bizarre idea that whole chunks of food enter your bloodstream.

To begin with, "intestinal permeability" is a real phenomenon (Eske, 2023). Basically, what happens is that water and nutrients pass through your intestine and into your blood while your entrails keep the harmful junk to themselves. This is a totally normal thing, a good thing, and one of the ways we extract nutrients and water from food. We need intestinal permeability.

The proposal around "leaky gut syndrome" is that there are cases in which this permeability goes totally off the rails. Furthermore, the proposal suggests that entire food particles, toxins, and bacteria enter the bloodstream, which results in you being unhealthy.

The symptoms of this alleged syndrome include bloating, chronic diarrhea (or constipation), fatigue, skin problems, and inflammation. Proponents also claim that it could be linked to autism.

So, let's tackle these one at a time.

First off, this is not a medically recognized diagnosis. Which, of course, does not mean it is not true, but there are several additional factors that might tip us off to its fictionality.

There is a lot of talk about "toxins" in the health and wellness community. Think of all the things you can buy, like that electrified water or whatever that is—the one you stick your feet in and it turns color? Anyway, that is supposed to pull toxins from your body. So is that electric blanket, and so are a whole bunch of other things.

The problem is, nothing much is ever said about these things other than that they are "toxins." What kind of toxin? Where do you get them from? What the heck does "toxin" even mean, anyway?

Second, I think we should be skeptical of a disease that is supposed to cause diarrhea *and* constipation. Call me crazy.

And finally, notice that "bacteria" are implicated. We know now that not all bacteria are bad for us. Some of them are good, necessary, or healthy. My feeling is that "bacteria" is used here as an emotional word. It is supposed to make you feel icky and gross, as opposed to giving you real information.

But most of all, come on. Whole food particles are entering the bloodstream.

Even a tiny air bubble in your blood can kill you. It will for sure give you a heart attack or a stroke and is considered a medical emergency. And air bubbles can burst! So really, even the tiniest particle of food in your blood would cause you to call an ambulance.

I used to work in factories when I was young. We would have these air hoses to clean off the machines after work because they would get dusted with steel particles and that weird matter that comes from welding. (I can't remember what it is called to save my life.)

Anyway, some people would use the air hoses to clean their clothes off at the end of the day. But the thing was, if you had a cut anywhere on you, the air hose would force air into your blood, which would cause it to move through your bloodstream.

What is the solution to this problem? If it ever happened—and thankfully it did not—we had to stab the air bubble with a pen or other sharp object. The idea was to force it to burst instead of letting it travel to a person's heart, where it might kill them.

So, I ask you: What are the odds that people have such leaky guts that food is just getting sucked into their bloodstream, and this is *not* killing them?

***

All of these myths and FAQs are part of a point I am trying to make.

There are always going to be wild claims around the subject of health. Old wives' tales, which is likely not the preferred term anymore, spread like wildfire. We hear something, we repeat it, they repeat it, and on it goes until a critical mass of people assume it is a fact.

Whether that is chewing gum sitting in your stomach for seven years or that bacteria are all bad for you, it does not matter. *Bullshit*, as a technical term meaning something that appears to be true but is not, is always present.

Unfortunately, the only way to counter bad information is with good information. And acquiring good information takes work. But since this is our health we are talking about, acquiring that good information is, of course, worth the price of admission.

I hope that this chapter has given us motivation to think about what bad information might look like. And then, I hope it has inspired us to want to look for the right information so that we can begin to take steps toward good health.

Alright. That about does it for the myths. Let's get to wrapping this thing up.

Conclusion

So here we are at the end of the line. We have been riding the train together for a while now. We had some laughs and shared a few moments. But now the train is slowing down, the station is coming into view through the window, and over the PA, we are being told to remain seated until the train has come to a complete stop.

Like all trips with other people, both long and short, there is no way of knowing ahead of time if either of us has made an impression on the other. For all I know, you might walk off the train, give your loved ones a big "I miss you" hug, and think, *God, that is the last time I ever talk to strangers on trains...*

But maybe some of what I have said here resonates with you. Maybe, at the very least, when you go out for dinner with the friends you have not seen in a long time—the ones you were riding the train into town to see—you will think for even just a split second about the food you order.

You might think, "There is a good to fair chance that this might make me sluggish, queasy, and ruin my mood. Maybe I should try something else."

And from there, you might tell that voice to shut up. That would be your prerogative, obviously. But maybe you will listen to that voice. And if that is the case, then I consider myself to have successfully performed my task.

But still, there may be some of you who are interested in doing this but who think it is too difficult. You might know that you do not take care of yourself very well and that this has started to affect your mental and physical health. But you may have such a habit of eating these kinds of sugary, not-good-for-gut-bacteria foods that you are not sure you can make the healthy choice. You might, you think, have come too far.

Well, then maybe I should tell you about my cousin Toby.

Toby was not what anyone would call "exceptional." Not that there was anything wrong with him either; he just never fooled anyone into thinking he was the next president or even a branch manager. He was a regular old, workaday type of guy, the kind with modest ambitions. He was the kind of guy who married his high school girlfriend.

When he was a teenager, he was not in bad shape. He did a lot of shop classes and that sort of thing, so he lifted machines around and lugged wood. He had a bit of a thing for beer but no more than any other teenager.

I would usually see him on holidays. And we would catch up, which was never a drawn-out conversation by any means. There was very little to say. He was working in one of the warehouses out of town; he had a girlfriend, and he was going to marry her—the works.

Then, one day, right around Easter, he came back a much, much larger man.

Right away, everyone took notice. It was awful, but how could we not? He had put on a serious amount of weight. And he knew that we knew, which of course, made it worse. You could tell he was hiding himself, turning to the side when he talked to everyone.

All his aunts, uncles, and cousins did the right thing and did not mention it—until, of course, he left. And then you know how people are. They expressed shock; they gossiped. All families are alike that way.

But I just wondered what the hell had happened. Was he depressed? Was he sick? How had he gained—no joke—45 pounds in the five months since I had seen him last?

As it turned out, what had happened to him was what happens to a lot of us. His metabolism had just bottomed out. When he was young, he could eat whatever he wanted. He did not have to think about it twice. Then he got older, and that part of him slowed down. Eventually, he could not eat whatever he wanted, but he had become so used to it that he didn't know how to stop; even once it became obvious he was gaining weight.

Unfortunately for him, the weight gain did not stop at 45 pounds. It went up to 60, which put him at about 255. And then he plateaued completely.

For years, he was that heavy. Eventually, it got to the point where we just got used to him being a big guy. We would see pictures of him when he was young and would kind of shake our heads at how things change, but that was that. He was the big brother in the family, and nobody even really noticed it anymore.

But, as I found out, he did.

You see, even as his weight became a fixture for us, it never got to be that way for him. As he told me years later, he struggled with it every single day. He could still see himself in his body, he said. He added that his real self was in there somewhere, and the extra stuff around him felt unreal.

At some point—I am not sure when exactly—he decided that it was time to change. Maybe it was a gradual thing, or maybe it came on suddenly. But he decided he did not like the way he looked, and he wanted to do something about it.

Now, it's not that nobody believed he could do it, necessarily. But he would bring it up at family functions that things were going to change for him. And I think everyone had the same reaction. They thought that if it would make him happy, then of course he should do it. But he had been this way for years. And he was, remember, somewhat unexceptional.

He was the kind of guy who was always fine with things the way they were. Until then, anyway. How would the guy who did, eventually, actually marry his high school sweetheart, who worked the same job he had worked since he graduated high school—how was that guy going to make the big changes necessary to turn his life around?

He must have seen it in our eyes. He must have known that we did not think he could pull it off. Because, as his wife Tracy told us later, he went at it like he had never gone at anything before.

First, he tried some of the fad diets. He tried Atkins and keto (which are the same, but whatever), and he tried the grapefruit diet and a few others. He would notice a bit of a change, and then usually, it would plateau, or he would go back to what he had been.

He saw some nutritionists. He bought a whole stack of books, even though he and Tracy did not have much money. He read and read, and at work, supposedly, all he would ever talk about was how bodies worked and what he needed to do to get to his goal weight.

Eventually, he felt like he'd hit his stride. He was shedding pounds, down to about 203 or thereabouts. He seemed confident and happy. He and Tracy were expecting their first around then, and he could not wait, as he said, "to bring some stern, hard-ass of a hockey player into this world."

But right after Tracy gave birth to their son Max, he hurt himself at work. He blew out his knee, lifting something beyond his capacity.

He had to spend a bit of time in the hospital. When he finally got home, he found himself immobile for a few months, which meant sitting on the couch. Which meant eating like he used to. Which meant, soon enough, that all of that weight came back.

And then some.

Now, I cannot imagine the level of defeat and frustration he must have felt. You could see it in him for about a year afterward—that he was tired. He would even crack jokes about how being a dad meant your body changed shape. He had resigned himself to not looking the way he had hoped.

But then he had a revelation. He said it happened while he was watching football. All these fellows were getting hammered by enormous guys, coming off the field limping and then running back on to do more damage and catch more balls.

And the thing is, he is a football fan. He knows the training and whatever else these guys take on. He has seen the videos where they talk about exercise and diet and what it takes to be in good enough shape to take a tackle by someone who is 300 pounds.

He had been going at it all wrong. The fad diet may have given him temporary weight loss. But he had not been exercising enough, which was why he had busted his knee. He was not an old man. And the weight that had wrecked his knee should not have been too much for him.

Maybe, then, the answer was way simpler than all these fad diets. Maybe it really did just come down to a healthy, balanced diet and exercise.

Over the next couple of years you could see the changes in him. He was eating plenty of vegetables and lots of fruit. He was going easy on red meat and eating whole grains.

And he was exercising. He would run three mornings a week. And do weights for three or four days. And that was just the start. Eventually, he would run five mornings a week and lift weights all those afternoons too.

Now, when you see him? He is a big fella. But it is muscle and fitness.

And more than that, it is his presence.

He is confident. Happy. He has three kids, and he can keep up with all of them. Sometimes, he even tires *them* out.

He and Tracy are so happy. He recently got a promotion. And as he puts it, he has never felt better in his life.

So, on the one hand, the reason why I have told you this is that Toby was not one of those Instagram fitness people who call you a pussycat for not trying to lift an entire truck over your head. Or who claim to work out three times every day before breakfast. He is just a regular guy who ran into some regular problems. And he solved it in the simplest way possible.

But the other reason is that, while I do not know this for a fact, I think we can see the results of everything we have talked about in his story.

Our guts are these amazing, hidden universes within us. They extend to every area of our bodies, affecting our feelings of wellness, our ability to fight disease, and even our mental health. Our guts, when they are in balance, help us digest food, which we need, but it makes us sick if we do not have the assistance of the bacteria that we have coevolved with to metabolize these things.

Toby's diet when he got big was what you would expect from most small-town men in the West. He liked his burgers and fries. He had hotdog BBQs every weekend. He enjoyed his beer.

And all of those things are fine and great—in moderation. The problem was that he overdid it. And his metabolism went squirrelly on him.

Our guts are partly responsible for our metabolism, no? Could that explain why it declined on him? Did he lose too much of the good bacteria to be able to digest these wild, Western foods?

What about his mental health? He became anxious and miserable. Part of that was self-image, no doubt. But could that not also have been because our guts are part of the process of making serotonin—the happy chemical?

And was gut health not at least part of the reason he is such a different person now?

Look, I have said before that I did not come here to make wild claims. I did not come here because I know how to change someone's life. I just know that this second brain of ours, this unseen universe within us, is responsible for so much of our health that not taking care of it and not considering it as part of our overall wellness is foolish.

By taking care of our gut health, we take care of ourselves. You have read the proof I have demonstrated for you. I think I have been convincing.

But hey, that is not for me to decide. Because, like I said, this is where we part ways. We have exited the train. My destination is to the left, and yours is to the right. We may never see each other again.

But if I have done my job here, then you will know that this unseen universe within us needs to be taken care of. And there is no doubt in my mind that you are more than capable of heeding this call.

Your health is within your grasp. Now, all you need to do is claim it.

Additional Resources

Books

All of the following can be found on Amazon:

Giulia Enders, Jill Enders. *Gut: The Inside Story of Our Body's Most Underrated Organ.* 2018.

Emeran Mayer. *The Mind-Gut Connection: How the Hidden Conversation Within Our Bodies Impacts Our Mood, Our Choices, and Our Overall Health.* 2018.

William Davis, M.D. *Super Gut: Reprogram Your Microbiome to Restore Health, Lose Weight, and Turn Back the Clock.* 2022.

Will Bulsiewicz. *Fiber Fueled: The Plant-Based Gut Health Program for Losing Weight, Restoring Your Health, and Optimizing Your Microbiome.* 2020.

Dr. Will Cole. *Gut Feelings: Healing the Shame-Fueled Relationship Between What You Eat and How You Feel.* 2023.

Articles

The "references" section of this book contains a number of articles, both scientific and popular. Without them this book would not have been possible.

Please consider consulting them for more detailed information. Many of their authors have written a number of other articles on these subjects also.

Remember, it is always better to get your information from the source. Scientific journals are your friend.

Wellness Experts

If this book has interested you, and you want to take the study and practice of wellness a step further, I recommend considering a wellness expert to help you along.

If you can, try to find a local dietitian to consult with for food- and diet-related matters. Also look into yoga instructors and gym memberships.

For meditation, there are a number of apps which I have used over the years. These provide guided meditations and should be considered indispensable:

Waking Up.
Calm.
Headspace.

Congratulations, Gut Health Campion!

You did it! You've reached the end of "Gut Wellness Simplified: Exploring the Unseen Universe Within Us," and we couldn't be prouder of your dedication to holistic well-being.

As you close this chapter, don't forget to grab your FREE 7-Day Gut Healing Meal Plan, and shopping list. It's not too late to supercharge your gut wellness journey with nourishing recipes and thoughtful guidance.

If you haven't already, scan the QR code below to access your downloadable PDF. Your gut health transformation starts here!

Remember, every step you take towards prioritising your gut wellness is a celebration of self-care and resilience. Embrace this moment and get ready to fuel your body, mind, and spirit with nourishing goodness.

Here's to a vibrant, thriving you and a future filled with boundless wellness! Thank you for being an inspiring champion of gut health.

Would you mind leaving a review? If you enjoyed this book, your feedback would mean the world to us and help others on their own gut wellness journeys.

Warm regards,

Olivia Rivers

References

Akkasheh, G., Huang, R., Wang, K., & Hu, J. (2016, August 6). *Effect of probiotics on depression: A systematic review and meta-analysis of randomized controlled trials.* PubMed. https://www.ncbi.nlm.nih.gov/pmc/articles/PMC4997396/

Campbell, K. (2020, March 2) *The science on gut microbiota and intestinal gas: Everything you wanted to know but didn't want to ask* ISAPP Science Blog. https://isappscience.org/the-science-on-gut-microbiota-and-intestinal-gas-everything-you-wanted-to-know-but-didnt-want-to-ask/

Carver-Carter, R. (2022, January 5). *Common gut health myths debunked.* Atlas Biomed Blog. https://atlasbiomed.com/blog/common-gut-health-myths-debunked/

Dix, M., and Klein, E. (2023, January 23). *Understanding gut health: Signs of an unhealthy gut and what to do about it.* Healthline. https://www.healthline.com/health/gut-health#improving-gut-health.

Eske, J. (2023, January 6). *What to know about leaky gut syndrome.* Medical News Today. https://www.medicalnewstoday.com/articles/326117. Accessed 19 September 2023.

Fick, L. (n.d.). *The magical medicine of bezoars*. HowStuffWorks. https://science.howstuffworks.com/life/biology-fields/magical-medicine-of-bezoars.htm.

Fu, J. Bonder, M., Carmen, Cenit, M., Tigchelaar, E., Maatman, A., Dekens, J., Brandsma, E., Marczynska, J., Imhann, F., Weersma, R., Franke, L., Poon, T., Xavier, R., Gevers, D., Hofker, M., Wijmenga, C., & Zhernakova, A. (2015, September 10). *The gut microbiome contributes to a substantial proportion of the variation in blood lipids*. Circulation Research, 117, (9), 817–824. https://doi.org/10.1161/circresaha.115.306807.

Jones, T. (2023, April 21). *Is it bad to eat before bed?* Healthline. https://www.healthline.com/nutrition/eating-before-bed#1

Kim, Y., Unno, T., Kim, B., & Park, M. (2020, January). *Sex differences in gut mictobiota*. PubMed. https://www.ncbi.nlm.nih.gov/pmc/articles/PMC6920072/

Kingsley, L. (2023, February 7). *The seesawing history of fad diets*. Smithsonian Magazine. https://www.smithsonianmag.com/innovation/the-seesawing-history-of-fad-diets-180981586/

Kostic AD., Gevers D., Siljander H., Vatanen T., Hyötyläinen T., Hämäläinen AM, Peet A., Tillmann V., Pöhö P, Mattila I., Lähdesmäki H., Franzosa EA., Vaarala O., de Goffau M., Harmsen H., Ilonen J., Virtanen SM., Clish CB., Orešič M., Huttenhower C., Knip M., DIABIMMUNE Study Group & Xavier RJ. (2015,

February 11). *The dynamics of the human infant gut microbiome in development and in progression toward type 1 diabetes.* PubMed. https://pubmed.ncbi.nlm.nih.gov/25662751/

Kristina, C. (2020, March 2). *The science on gut microbiota and intestinal gas: Everything you wanted to know but didn't want to ask.* International Scientific Association for Probiotics and Prebiotics (ISAPP). https://isappscience.org/the-science-on-gut-microbiota-and-intestinal-gas-everything-you-wanted-to-know-but-didnt-want-to-ask/ Accessed 19 September 2023.

Kubala, J. (2019, March 6). *Is gluten bad for you? A critical look.* Healthline. https://www.healthline.com/nutrition/is-gluten-bad

Marshall, B., & Adams, P. (2008, November). *Helicobacter pylori: A nobel pursuit.* PubMed. https://www.ncbi.nlm.nih.gov/pmc/articles/PMC2661189/

McDermott, A. (2017, March 21). *Everything you should know about coffee enemas.* Healthline. https://www.healthline.com/health/coffee-enema?utm_source=ReadNext. Accessed 19 September 2023.

McPhillips, D. (2022, October 5). *90% of US adults say the United States is experiencing a mental health crisis.* CNN. https://edition.cnn.com/2022/10/05/health/cnn-kff-mental-health-poll-wellness/index.html.

Miller, A. (2018, April 30). *Five things to know about inflammation and depression.* Psychiatric Times. https://www.psychiatrictimes.com/view/five-things-know-about-inflammation-and-depression

Moore, W. (2009) *John Hunter (1728-1793).* The James Lind Library. https://www.jameslindlibrary.org/articles/john-hunter-1728-93/

Pratt, E. (2018, September 24). *Research says exercise also improves your gut bacteria.* Healthline. https://www.healthline.com/health-news/exercise-improves-your-gut-bacteria

Reddy, D. (2022, May 16). *Gut health for women: Care for and feed your second brain.* WakeMed Voices. https://wakemedvoices.com/2022/05/gut-health-for-women-the-care-and-feeding-of-your-second-brain/Accessed 19 September 2023.

Ridaura, V., Faith, J., Rey, F., Cheng, J., Duncan, A., Kau, A., Griffin, N., Lombard, V., Henrissat, B., Bain, J., Muehlbauer, M., Ilkayeva, O., Semenkovich, C., Funai, K., Hayashi, D., Lyle, B., Martini, M., Ursell, L., Clemente, J., Treuren, W., Walters, W., Knight, R., Newgard, C., Heath, A., & Gordon, J. (2013, September 6). *Gut microbiota from twins discordant for obesity modulate metabolism in mice.* Science (New York, N.Y.), 341, (6150). https://doi.org/10.1126/science.1241214

Robertson, R. (2023, April 3). *How does your gut microbiome impact your overall health?* Healthline. https://www.healthline.com/nutrition/gut-microbiome-and-health

Robertson, R. (2023, July 31). *The gut-brain connection: How it works and the role of nutrition.* Healthline. https://www.healthline.com/nutrition/gut-brain-connection#TOC_TITLE_HDR_5

Santos-Longhurst, (2018, July 31). *How long does gum take to digest?* Healthline. https://www.healthline.com/health/how-long-does-gum-take-to-digest

Singh, R, Chang, H., Yan, D., Lee, K., Ucmak, D., Wong, K., Abrouk, M., Farahnik, B., Nakamura, M., Zhu, T., Bhutani, T., & Liao, W. (2017, April 8). *Influence of diet on the gut microbiome and implications for human health.* Journal of Translational Medicine, 15, (1). https://doi.org/10.1186/s12967-017-1175-y

Solgar. (2023, May 23). *The 10 best gut-healthy foods for women.* Solgar. https://www.solgar.com/blog/nutrition/gut-health-foods-women/

The Nutrition Professionals. (2022, June 13). *The link between gut health & hormones explained.* The Nutrition Professionals. https://nutritionpro.net/the-link-between-gut-health-hormones-explained/

WebMD Editorial Contributors. (2023, September 11). *What is a bezoar?* WebMD. www.webmd.com/digestive-disorders/what-is-a-bezoar

White, A. (2023, October 19). *8 ways to do a natural colon cleanse at home.* Healthline. https://www.healthline.com/health/natural-colon-cleanse

Printed in Great Britain
by Amazon